Recovering and Healing
After The Narcissist

Recovering and Healing After The Narcissist

DISCOVERING YOUR TRUE SELF

Linda Martinez-Lewi, Ph.D.

Printed in the United States of America

First Printing, 2015

ISBN 978-0-578-84380-3

Library of Congress Control Number: 2021902146

Surrey Publishing

www.thenarcissistinyourlife.com

Dedication

For Peter whose love, inspiration and devotion
Through every weather has helped me to grow and evolve
…The words and the music.

Table of Contents

Acknowledgements

I AM DEEPLY GRATEFUL TO artist Andrea Bodet, whose perceptive insights and creative support contributed to the structure and flow of this book.

Deep appreciation to Charlotte Armstrong, the noted suspense writer, who was my intellectual and literary mentor. I learned from her about the territories of the unconscious mind, the complexities of human nature, the mysteries of the creative process and the discipline required to write professionally.

Preface

HEALING IS A NATURAL LIFE process. The human body is miraculous in its capacity to heal when we provide it with the necessary nutrients, healthy practices and environment. The psyche and mind of those who have suffered and endured the pain of narcissistic abuse can be restored to wholeness.

There are many pathways to recovery following a relationship with a narcissistic spouse, mother, father or sibling. In the aftermath of your relationship with a narcissist, you can recover and thrive. This is accomplished through essential practices of self-care that activate and instill the healing and recovery process.

I was inspired to write this book by the life experiences of my readers and clients who spoke and wrote to me about the psychological and emotional devastation they endured as a result of their relationships with narcissists. Those who live in the aftermath of the narcissist experience deep pain; they feel desperate, frightened, angry, confused, exhausted, lost and alone. The purpose of this book is to provide you with the specific tools of a self-care practice for recovering your true self, deep inner peace, psychological and emotional balance and your unique creative gifts.

Your journey of recovery begins now. You seek and will discover the true self, the great healer that restores, comforts, renews and guides you through all of your days.

CHAPTER 1

Leaving the Narcissist: Your Healing Begins

Finding the center of strength within ourselves
is in the long run the best contribution we
can make to our fellow men. One person with
indigenous inner strength exercises a great
calming effect ... among people around him.

—ROLLO MAY

Because the development of inner calm
and energy happens completely within
and isn't dependent on another person ...
we begin to feel a resourcefulness and
independence that is quite beautiful...

—SHARON SALZBERG

WHEN WE SEPARATE OURSELVES FROM the narcissist,
our consciousness expands and deepens. The true self

grows without impingements, creates without boundaries, expresses feelings openly and thinks with a spacious mind. Those who put seeking the true self uppermost in their lives receive a great boon—the hero's journey. Freeing yourself from the narcissist who took so much of your life is a major step toward individuation. Taking this journey you dis-identify from the narcissist and rediscover your life's work—becoming your authentic self.

I address this book to those who are experiencing emotional and psychological pain, confusion and anxiety in the aftermath of their destructive relationships with narcissists. My purpose is to help those who have been victimized to recognize that they are not to blame for this cruel, unwarranted emotional devastation and that they can heal fully.

QUESTIONS FROM VICTIMS OF NARCISSISTIC PERSONALITIES

In this book I am responding to questions and painful life stories from those who are or have been victimized by narcissistic personalities. My first book, *Freeing Yourself from the Narcissist in Your Life,* has been very well received. It introduces readers to the narcissistic personality disorder in depth. This book is a guide for those who are working to heal from these toxic relationships and provides essential strategies for rediscovering their true selves.

I have spoken to spouses, ex-spouses, children and siblings of narcissistic personalities and others who continue to suffer from the cruel aftermath these individuals leave in their wake. Each life story is unique with an underlying theme: How can I heal myself from narcissistic abuse and regain my psychological, emotional, creative and spiritual freedom?

The following is a composite of questions communicated to me by those who have been emotionally and psychologically battered by the narcissists in their lives:

- *My husband divorced me several months ago. I still feel tied to him. How do I stop the pain and put my life back together?*
- *I have a narcissistic mother who never loved me. I was her servant. Should I break off contact with her?*
- *My husband/wife constantly lied and cheated on me. How can I make the break and heal from these betrayals?*
- *I have married and divorced two narcissistic husbands. I'm still drawn to these lethal charmers. How can I protect myself and not repeat this destructive pattern?*
- *I am still trying to heal after divorcing my narcissistic wife/husband. I suffer from chronic insomnia and feel defeated.*
- *I have deep emotional scars years after breaking up with a narcissistic boyfriend. I don't think I will ever love anyone again.*
- *I have been the victim of my narcissistic family. My mother, sister and brother scapegoated me all of my life.*

> *How can I heal from the emotional pain that I feel every day? I feel haunted by their cruelty and hatefulness.*
> * *I am physically and emotionally exhausted after a bitter divorce. I've lost a piece of myself. How can I feel hopeful again?*

These questions have answers and positive outcomes for those who seek healing, personal individuation and growth after their relationships with narcissists.

CHRISTINA'S STORY

A client, Christina, came to therapy after going through the ordeal of a complex and painful divorce from Steve, her narcissistic husband of fifteen years. Christina sacrificed herself seeking Steve's love and approval. A classic narcissist, Steve was incapable of being fully human. The ultimate proof was his complete lack of empathy, constant assertion of his superiority and chronic lying, deception and verbal abuse. The harder Christina worked at the marriage, the more cruelly she was treated.

Understanding the psychodynamics in Christina's family of origin is revealing. Christina's mother, Allison, a classic narcissist, was emotionally distant from her daughter. There was no hugging, no emotional closeness, no empathy. Christina's father, a workaholic, was absent for most of his daughter's childhood and adolescence. As a young woman, Christina searched for the perfect man who would complete her. She met Steve, a confident, handsome high achiever, who fulfilled all of her wishes in a husband. Soon after the wedding, Christina became aware of the real Steve beneath the smooth, irresistible persona. She was exposed to his ugly, enraged, controlling side. Christina was shocked and disturbed by the new Steve but was determined to make the marriage work. She was intimidated by Steve and obeyed him, putting every effort into becoming the perfect woman he expected. She told herself that if she were more patient and understanding then Steve would love her.

After many painful verbal skirmishes, Christina realized that Steve was not going to change. She could not cope with his volcanic rage, lack of empathy and deceitfulness. She was psychologically and physically worn out. She reached out to a close friend who referred her to an excellent therapist. Christina began the process of grieving over her marriage. She cried often as she let go of Steve but found she was able to deal with the realization that they would never be together again.

Christina formed a strong therapeutic alliance with her therapist, who validated and supported Christina throughout the divorce. During the therapeutic process, Christina began to recognize her psychological pattern of repetition. She was the daughter of a narcissistic mother who was incapable of giving love. Christina had survived her cold, critical mother and absent father. In Steve she had found the "perfect husband," another narcissist who was hypercritical and dismissed her value as an individual.

Christina researched the narcissistic personality disorder. She recognized distinct characterological similarities between her narcissistic mother and her husband. She moved forward with the divorce. She practiced quieting her mind through meditation. As part of her healing, Christina severed ties with her narcissistic mother and absent father. After a lot of consistent work and commitment to healing, Christina is leading life on her terms as a separate, growing individual.

PURPOSE OF THIS BOOK

This book is written for those who have experienced narcissistic abuse from spouses, ex-spouses, parents, siblings and other family members. It is a guide to recovery of the true self, that part of you that is spontaneous, creative, spiritual, and intuitive, and has no limitations.

Chapter One defines the narcissist as an individual who suffers from a severe personality disorder that is characterized by extreme self-absorption, lack of empathy, limited conscience, deception and an incapacity for emotional intimacy.

Chapter Two addresses the lifelong process of psychological separation and individuation that is an integral part of healing from narcissists. The qualities of the individuated self are described.

Chapter Three focuses on breaking up regressive, self-limiting, psychological patterns of repetitive thinking, feelings and actions. The compulsion to repeat is part of an unbroken cycle in relationships with the narcissistic personality. Breaking up these repetitions frees the individual to take the initiative to choose partners who are capable of genuine love and emotional intimacy.

Chapter Four introduces an essential tool of personal transformation, daily writing practice. Writing is one of the most powerful ways of freeing yourself from the psychological oppression you suffered under the narcissist.

Chapter Five invites readers to tap into their creativity. The shadow archetype, introduced by psychoanalyst Carl Jung, is described. Working with the shadow deepens and expands the limitless capacity to create. Experiencing nature in its glorious forms is an integral part of the healing process. Music's mystical flow bathes us in a reality of perpetual beauty.

Chapter Six explores the rich territories of friendships and how they heal psychological and emotional wounds. Within the security and comfort of a genuine friendship, we are not alone and are kindly understood. Friends give us the courage to realize that our visions can be realities.

Chapter Seven describes and explains the meditation process. Meditation is one of the most powerful and effective tools for shifting to clearer consciousness. After many years of living in fight-or-flight mode with the narcissist, meditation activates the relaxation response.

Chapter Eight assists you in awakening and activating your true self. An essential part of this process is using the breath to experience calmness and inner security. In this chapter, there is an exploration of several ways of accessing the parasympathetic nervous system through acupuncture, the healing power of the unconscious, the creation of Blue Zone Islands of creativity and calm and the experience of the healing moment, where souls meet and healing takes place.

Chapter Nine is the Recovery Journal, a guide and companion for keeping track of your healing and growth process.

IDENTIFYING THE NARCISSISTIC PERSONALITY

Narcissistic personality disorders are characterized by extreme self-absorption, lack of empathy, ruthlessness, incapacity for emotional intimacy, volcanic rage, chronic lying, deceit and exploitation. Narcissists don't form genuine relationships. They treat others like objects from whom they obtain narcissistic supplies: adulation, praise, professional and social status, monetary gain and worldly power. The narcissist believes he is superior to others. He has an overriding sense of self-entitlement, thinking he can have whatever and whomever he wants because he is special and irresistible. Each person the narcissist meets is assessed as an opportunity for him to climb and reach the heady air of the highest peaks of success. The narcissist lacks a conscience; his sense of right and wrong is determined by how clever he is at not being exposed or punished for his unethical, immoral and illegal behaviors.

For the narcissist, everyone is disposable; one person is interchangeable with another. He lures and seduces each one with his magnetic charm and takes possession and control of their identities, their thoughts and feelings, their lives. After he has fully exploited their emotional vulnerability, blocked their creativity and put them in financial jeopardy, the narcissist hastily exits. He has neither a memory nor one scintilla of concern about the victims of his psychological crimes. Smelling the sweet aroma of victory, this conquistador grabs his sword and moves confidently forward. As part of fulfilling his grandiose vision, the narcissist charms a new circle of people who will play their assigned parts as adoring followers and provide him with obedience, blind loyalty and selfless service.

The narcissist is secretly envious of those whom he views as superlative winners. A dirty fighter, the narcissist uses malignant lies and innuendoes to destroy the professional and personal reputations of his competitors and bête noires. The narcissist is secretly paranoid, experiencing an overwhelming fear that others will harm him. He fiercely protects himself from real and imagined enemies.

Beneath the elaborate mask of a grandiose false self, the narcissist unconsciously experiences a deep, intractable psychological emptiness.

The hallmark of the narcissistic personality disorder is a complete lack of empathy, the capacity to put oneself emotionally in the place of another. Narcissists are great method actors who affect a persuasive pseudo-empathy that is brilliantly performed.

LIFE IN THE AFTERMATH OF THE NARCISSIST

Leaving the psychological imprisonment of the narcissist is a powerful motivator for separating and evolving toward your real self. This process is challenging and painful, but ultimately very rewarding. Initially, there are feelings of confusion and disorientation. You have invested so much of yourself in the relationship, identified so strongly with the narcissist and his empty promises, that it can be difficult to distinguish psychologically who you are as a separate person.

Some victims are in a state of shock, discovering that the narcissist has stolen many years from their lives. When they realize they were never truly loved, those who have chosen to share their lives with these treacherous individuals go through periods of denial, dismay, rage, confusion and grief. The narcissist leaves chaos and destruction in his wake in the form of lies, betrayals, financial reverses and psychological and physical health issues. The litany of sins perpetrated by the narcissist is long and cuts deeply into the psyches of his victims.

In separating from the narcissist, many go through a grieving process. Having tried multiple times to save the relationship, the narcissist's victim is weary, frightened, exhausted and hanging by a narrowing thread. Many spouses and ex-spouses find it hard to give up the fight; they are instilled with the idea of preserving a marriage and family and feel a deep obligation to do this despite the emotional cost to them. Some victims of narcissists obsess about how they could have behaved differently to help the narcissist change; however, changing a narcissist is clinically improbable since narcissistic personality is a highly fixed psychological disorder.

Those who are married to narcissists and precipitously discarded are flooded with disbelief. They say to themselves, *This couldn't be happening. I am imagining it. It can't be true.* One moment they believe they have a happy marriage; the next, they have been told that it is over, that they no longer have a life with their spouses of many years and that their families are permanently divided. Some spouses use every method to beg their narcissistic partner to reconsider. They don't realize that the narcissist knew long ago that he was going to throw them overboard. They could no longer provide him with essential narcissistic supplies. Their brightness had faded. They were a burden he had to dispose of quickly. Coming on the heels of the shock and denial is a searing pain to the heart.

The next step is acknowledging and working through the rage. The compulsion to strike back, to injure the narcissist, is strong. Some spouses have great difficulty moving through this phase; they are angry with themselves for being martyred by such a malevolent human being. Other spouses and ex-spouses reprimand themselves: *How could I possibly have swallowed so many lies and danced to his psychological choreography for so long?*

As the rage subsides, some individuals feel very alone, without a rudder or life focus. Many ex-spouses find that quality psychotherapy helps them express their feelings openly with an excellent listener and develop a therapeutic alliance of trust. This allows them to clarify where they stand in their lives and how they will proceed in the future.

CHECKING YOUR PROGRESS:

Healing from the narcissist begins with small steps. Give yourself credit for all of your efforts. There are no mistakes. You are growing and evolving each day.

- Make a list of what you did **for yourself** this week.
- Envision your future. Spontaneously write down what you are seeing without editing.

- What are you noticing inside yourself that indicates the narcissist is no longer uppermost in your thoughts and feelings?
- How are you expressing creative capacities?
- What are you learning about yourself as a unique individual?

CHAPTER 2

Separation/Individuation: How We Become Individuals

Like a seed growing into a tree, life unfolds
stage by stage ... only if he treads the path
bravely and flings himself into life, fearing
no struggle and no exertion ... will he
mature his personality more fully ...

—JOLANDE JACOBI

Knowing your own darkness is the best method
for dealing with the darknesses of other people.

—CARL GUSTAV JUNG

WHEN THE NUCLEUS OF A single human sperm cell
penetrates the nucleus of a ripe egg, the ovum, fertil-
ization occurs. The product of this union is a zygote.
The zygote, the essential core of human beginnings, is

formed, and the dynamic, miraculous process of creating a human being is underway. Each body system—cardiovascular, lymphatic, digestive, endocrine, muscular, nervous, reproductive, respiratory, excretory and skeletal—grows and interconnects in an unfolding fullness to create a separate, unique individual.

At birth, the baby separates from physical symbiosis with the mother and breathes on his own for the first time. The newborn lives in an oceanic union with mother. For him there is no *me or not me,* only *mother and me.* Gradually, over the first months of life, physical and psychological separation begins. At two to three months the baby experiences the first steps toward recognizing that he is distinct from his mother, distinguishing psychological and physical boundaries between his mother and himself. The infant is aware of a growing separateness from her; his sense of self is unfolding. He is becoming an "I" and she is becoming a "you." Between the ages of six months and a year and a half the young child is constantly experimenting: learning to sit up independently, to crawl and scoot, to bring himself to a standing position, to learn how to fall and get up again and again, to walk unsteadily and finally to move with his feet grounded on the earth. The child experiences excitement and joy as he discovers that he can move all by himself. Being able to walk away from his mother, he recognizes that he moves independently through space using his own power and purpose. One of the most beautiful scenes to watch is a very young child practicing his walking. As he gains more skill and strength, he runs as fast as he can with great abandon. Along with the achievement of many physical capacities, the child's psyche and mind is expanding.

BECOMING AN INDIVIDUAL

The stages of the individuated self unfold in the growing child. The beginnings of speech—repeated sounds, words, phrases, then sentences—flow through the young child. His thoughts and feelings are transformed into words, a powerful form of communication that reinforces his unique identity. Expression through speech is part of activating the child's gifts of imagination, creative self-expression as well as the expanded ability to give voice to his feelings. The constant practice of speech by the infant is truly remarkable. I have heard children repeating words and phrases as if they were practicing intricate notes on a scale. Their efforts and perseverance to master the spoken word is a marvel. The young child's capacities for play and a vibrant sense of humor ripen along with the unique creativity that he brings to every activity in his life.

As the child grows and matures, his inner and outer worlds are expanded and enriched by multitudes of influences within his family, friends, community and innumerable points of human contact. The child's exposure and acquaintance with the natural world combined with his private perceptions, thoughts, feelings and insights add pieces to the mosaic of this dynamic living individual.

As the child develops, he explores the outer world beyond his home environment. At school he has opportunities to develop his mental capacities, to think independently and creatively and to learn about the complexities of social interactions with friends and fellow students.

During adolescence, an often turbulent time, the pubescent experiments with greater personal freedom, emerging sexuality, evolving identity, social skills and expanding his intellectual and creative capacities. The stormy period of adolescence is an integral part of the individuation process.

Parents who constantly tell you that they have "good kids," meaning that there are no problems, ugly scenes, arguments, resistance or rage on the part of their children are either lying to you or concealing the truth from themselves.

The "good kid" focuses on pleasing his parents, emulating their thinking processes and behavioral patterns rather than becoming his real self. This child is too intimidated and controlled by the iron will of the parent to think and feel for himself, and, as a result, individuation, the process of becoming an authentic person, is stalled. Many parents view their children through rosy lenses and want to think they are raising a perfect "kid" because it reflects well on them. As a result, some "perfect kids" develop a false self and become budding narcissists.

There are serious psychological issues that arise from not separating and individuating out of the parental mold. Despite many external achievements, like superior grades, smooth social skills, athletic talent and creative gifts, the young adult remains unconsciously tied to his parents' ambitions for him rather than dis-identifying from mother and father to become his unique self.

The passage of adolescence is not supposed to be smooth and easy. It is essential for the child to take the necessary psychological steps away from the parent. During this time, the parents stand back and watch the young person they love move in increments to reach adulthood. The adolescent and young adult tests himself each time he crosses one of life's thresholds. There are many rickety wind-swept bridges of every design, length, age and condition that adolescents and young adults traverse.

We move through complex, painful, frightening and mysterious transitions throughout our lives. Each transit point presents an opportunity to individuate or stagnate and regress. The process of individuation is always waiting for us to say: "Yes, I will move forward, heal and become whole."

QUALITIES OF THE INDIVIDUATED SELF

We are born in complete dependence and vulnerability. Within us are the developmental seeds for individuation, a word that describes the growing edge of a strong, solid person who will flourish, expand and deepen. We work at the process of individuation throughout our lives. Opportunities for accelerating individuation often occur at times of psychological duress and life crises. Our pain, desperation and past regressive, repetitive, failed choices can awaken and inspire us to enter the waters of the river of change. This process, along with the hard, persevering work we do with ourselves, leads to psychological freedom.

Hold the reins of life firmly in your hands but loosely enough to maneuver its unexpected and mysterious terrains. To use a metaphor from fine horsemanship, the good rider uses his body, seat and legs to control his horse. Proper use of the reins is essential to the excellent horseman. Fine riders barely move their arms and upper bodies; they glide smoothly in rhythm with the movements of the horse. They communicate mainly with their seat: the buttocks, inner thighs, calves and ankles.

Like a rider trains to achieve good form, you work all of your life on becoming an individual. Your practice prepares you for the journey. As you move forward, your center, your psychological core, holds steady and strong.

Those who don't develop an independent sense of self tend to marry someone who controls, manipulates, deceives and demeans them. Often this partner is a narcissist. It is not unusual for a woman or man to marry more than one narcissist if they have grown up with narcissistic parents. They return to familiar pain. Breaking this destructive repetition cycle is essential to developing one's full psychological, creative, emotional and mental capacities.

INDEPENDENT THINKING: RESPECTING YOUR OWN PERCEPTIONS

You've heard of the terrible twos, that time when the child begins to assert himself, much to the consternation of his parents. This is a normal developmental process. The child is working toward psychological independence and self-initiating patterns of thinking, feeling and behavior.

Children who grew up with one or more narcissistic parents were never allowed to express their own feelings and thoughts or share their dreams and ambitions without ridicule. They were molded into living puppets ready to do the narcissistic parent's bidding. Growing up, these children believed their thinking was distorted and misguided. In some cases, narcissistic parents told their children they were bad kids or even crazy. As a result, many children of narcissists adopted the model set by their abusive parents and, to this day, doubt their own perceptions and feelings. Adults who grew up emotionally constricted remain numb and frozen. It isn't surprising that many of these individuals marry narcissists who indoctrinate them once more, repeating the brainwashing that was perpetrated on them as children.

As you heal from your narcissistic family or the dissolution of your marriage to a narcissist, you are released from mental and psychological imprisonment. Some victims of narcissistic abuse benefit from excellent psychotherapy and the practice of healing modalities such as daily self-care, gentle hatha yoga with emphasis on the breath and a form of meditation that quiets the nervous system, activating feelings of inner peace and well being.

Intuition is an invaluable life gift. Most of us override our intuition and argue with it. We have doubts about knowledge that comes to us so quickly. Despite our mistrust, intuition is a powerful guiding force. Every time I have turned away and sidestepped an intuitive message, I have made a big mistake. Intuition has velocity, momentum and deep penetration beneath the layers of the conscious thinking mind. It cuts through our ego barriers and comes through clear, sharp and true.

STILLING THE MIND THROUGH MEDITATION

'The Soul loves to meditate, for in contact with the Spirit lies its greatest joy..."
—Paramahansa Yogananda

When you begin to practice meditation, be patient with yourself. Meditation is a personal process. Don't judge yourself based on the way you feel when you are meditating. You will be distracted: Many thoughts swirl through your mind; you cycle into different moods and feelings; your back cramps, your nose itches; you are pulled by your emotions— fear, sadness, regret, anger, guilt, and envy. The quality, quantity and subjects of these distractions vary each time. Each meditation is valuable and unique, never to be repeated again.

Consistency is the most important component for developing a meditation practice. There is a powerful carryover effect as your meditations accumulate throughout the months and years. Meditation becomes a habit, a ritual of your day. If you forget to meditate, resume your practice regardless of how much time has elapsed. I have learned after many years that it is not the length of meditation that matters; it is your intention and taking action. A meditation of just a few minutes, even one or two minutes, can be very meaningful. Begin by settling yourself as comfortably as possible. Take a slow deep breath through the nose, hold one or two counts at the top, exhale slowly through the mouth. The exhalation should be longer than the inhalation because the exhaled breathing activates the parasympathetic nervous system.

Some meditations are choppy. You are making the effort, but thoughts, feelings and sensations flood your mind. As you recognize that you have gone on a mental detour, bring yourself back with the observation of your breath.

After you have been practicing for a while, you will begin to experience moments of living, dynamic peace. It may stay with you briefly, come and go, or take its place inside of you. Each person has a different experience. The spirit finds its special way into your mind and heart, using a language that speaks to you alone.

Your meditation practice and your intuitive gifts grow alongside and complement one another. Being highly intuitive becomes a part of your daily life experience.

CHECKING YOUR PROGRESS:

- What insights have you received through your intuition?
- What are some of your creative gifts?
- Name two life dreams you wish to fulfill.
- How are you celebrating your separate, authentic self?

CHAPTER 3

Breaking Cycles of Repetition: Changing Life Patterns

> The Buddha gave conditioned existence a name...
> Samsara is the Sanskrit word that describes
> the wheel of suffering that we perpetuate by
> doing the same thing time and time again.
>
> —LAMA SURYA DAS

> A thing which has not been understood inevitably
> reappears; like an unlaid ghost, it cannot rest until
> the mystery has been resolved and the spell broken.
>
> —SIGMUND FREUD

THE COMPULSION TO REPEAT

The concept of repetition has been a source of clinical interest to me for many years. As I observe individuals I ask myself: Why do we repeat the same destructive emotional, psychological and mental patterns year after year, decade after decade? What is the force, the psychological gravity that imprisons and constricts many individuals from leading productive, loving and creative lives? Why do we cause ourselves such pain or inflict it upon others? Why do we waste our potential as we spiral repeatedly into the rut of another repetitive sequence? Like a dancer that cannot pause, unable to stop despite nausea and dizziness, many of us are constantly pirouetting from one interpersonal or business disaster to the next.

The negative effects of dealing with a narcissist help explain these repetitive cycles. Maintaining a marital or familial relationship with a narcissist is very difficult, if not impossible. Since their personality structure is fixed and they believe they are perfect, your role with them is limited to being on the receiving end of their unconscious projections. These take innumerable forms: volcanic rage, delusional accusations, vindictive threats and elaborate lies. You find yourself reeling from overwhelming cycles of abuse that you cannot stop. Your life becomes a series of ongoing crises that deleteriously affect your mental, emotional and psychological health.

The compulsion to repeat is ever-present. If you were raised in a narcissistic family, it is not unusual for you to be attracted to and marry narcissistic men and women. An individual who has been victimized in a chaotic, painful first marriage to a narcissist will often repeat this pattern with a second or even third spouse.

Unconsciously repeating the same destructive psychological scenarios makes us unable to recognize our true emotions. We are suffering and can't acknowledge it, sick and denying it, furious and burying it. The original wounds of childhood have made us psychologically and spiritually numb to the truth of our core life experiences. When the slumber of denial becomes chronic, we find it increasingly difficult to rouse ourselves, to awaken and realize that we are trapped in a vortex of repetition that is keeping us from evolving as individuals.

ROOTS OF REPETITION: CHILDHOOD TRAUMA AND DEPRIVATION

Childhood trauma is a deep and chronic wounding of the self. It blunts psychological growth, personal creativity and the capacity to trust another human being. Trauma has many faces. It is psychologically destabilizing, physically weakening and emotionally distressing. If trauma becomes chronic, the child exists in a painful state of hyper-vigilance, free-floating anxiety and the incapacity to trust himself and others. The traumatized child takes different survival routes depending on his temperament, disposition and emotional and psychological sensitivity. He can numb himself, become steel-hard, tough and uncaring, or compartmentalize his inner life.

The survival tactics we develop become ingrained into us. Like a familiar song that spontaneously reprises in our minds, distinct patterns of thoughts, feelings, memories, fantasies and wishes emerge. Observing more closely, we discover intricate patterns of repetition. Most people continue to listen and respond to the old family life song first heard in childhood. The pitch varies, the instruments change, the vocalist is new, the venue is different, but the core message still resonates. The same unproductive and destructive psychological patterns of repetition that keep many individuals stuck and immobilized remain intact.

Repetition is an effort on the part of the psyche to shake off our delusions, to awaken us to the truth of our lives. When we work to become consciously aware of our psychological, emotional and behavioral repetitions, we are evolving and moving toward freedom and individuation.

The destructive life repetitions that we engage in are innumerable and particular to each individual. They are found in a repeated cycle of returning to narcissistic individuals who injure us emotionally and psychologically. It is surprising, but often the child that was raised in a narcissistic family with narcissistic parents and siblings returns to this environment that created his greatest suffering by marrying a narcissistic personality.

UNREMEMBERED AND UNFORGETTABLE

In human existence nothing is truly forgotten. Every experience we have ever had, from the most minute and remote to the truly epic, is recorded in every cell of our bodies, imprinted on mind, body and psyche. It is preserved in a living form that we do not recognize consciously. The assaults and abandonments that have been "forgotten" by their victims operate in the recesses of the unconscious; they remain active there and insinuate themselves into every aspect of our lives. "Forgotten" events inhabit dreams that reoccur.

Unprocessed trauma that has gone deeply into the unconscious is expressed in a variety of ways. In some cases it is projected onto others through rage, suspicions, accusations and threats. This is the case with a narcissistic personality, a false self who believes he is untouchable and superior. The narcissist uses others as receptacles to dispose of his virulent feelings of self-loathing, paranoia and envy. If you are the child, sibling or spouse of one of these individuals, you have been on the receiving end of this constant psychic fire. You are the perennial target of the full fury of this abuse.

We carry with us into adulthood the survival mechanisms we used as young children. These psychological defenses cause mental amnesia of the traumatic events that occurred during our early years and beyond. Some people experience significant gaps in memory. In many cases, absence of recollection is caused by crushing blows to the psychic structure that took place during the earliest years. In an effort to ward off highly painful events, some children create idealized "memories" of their mother, father and family environment.

In every family constellation there are secrets, betrayals, cruelties, verbal and emotional assaults and favoritisms. The glossy landscape of an idyllic childhood is a fabrication the parents foster to ward off and deny the ugly painful truth.

Growing up with narcissistic parental rejection, emotional abandonment and forceful psychological manipulation has severe consequences on a child's trust in himself and his emotional stability. The young child doesn't understand what has happened to him. In place of this understanding, a psychological numbing occurs that can result in a "forgetting." These assaults on the psyche are so severe that they cannot be consciously perceived as real. Traumas that occur very early and are chronically repeated have the most severe effects on the growth and progression of the real self.

No deprivation or cruelty perpetrated on a child simply disappears. Trauma returns in the language of dreams, addictions, obsessions, anxieties, mood disorders, physical illness and dissociative disorders. Unconscious repetitions of trauma are corrosive and debilitating, afflicting some victims for a lifetime.

The agony of maternal deprivation is one of the most wrenching human experiences. A child who is neglected, unprotected, dismissed or forgotten never feels safe. He cannot trust his own mind, nor can he express genuine emotion. His inner world is one of deadened inertness. Some clients describe this state to me as "being nonexistent."

The brilliant psychoanalyst Leonard Shengold, M.D., describes the horrific experiences the young child endures: "To abuse or neglect a child, to deprive the child of a separate identity, is to commit 'soul murder.'" Dr. Shengold believes that deprivation can be more traumatizing to a child than abuse. The child endures the absence, a piercing maternal void in the deep recesses of his psyche. Often these mothers are narcissistic and fully engrossed in satisfying their desires and wishes with total disregard for their child. For the narcissistic mother, the child is a source of narcissistic supply to inflate her ego or a burden and a nuisance that must be discarded.

The narcissistic mother's callousness and extreme self-involvement leave her children without any form of emotional and psychological sustenance. Mother is an empty lap with no arms for embracing, no warmth for protection, no steadiness for emotional security, no gesture of tenderness. She is a bottomless void. Narcissistic mothers throw their children to the winds of fate to capriciously decide where they will land and whether they will psychologically live or die.

Some narcissistic mothers fool those around them with their pseudo-solicitousness about their children's needs. This is cleverly designed to present their kids as a perfect reflection of themselves. They are obsessed with projecting the profile of a superior parent. The narcissistic mother makes certain that photographs are taken that display maternal devotion. In the neighborhood and the wider community, she is labeled as an exemplary parent, a "supermom."

In his book *Soul Murder,* Dr. Shengold presents a psychobiography of the great writer Rudyard Kipling, explaining how psychologically crushing events of his childhood were "an attempt at soul murder."

Rudyard was born in India and lived like a little prince in his native land until the age of six. At that time, the family moved to England. Without warning his parents surreptitiously left their six-year-old son Rudyard and three-year-old daughter Alice with highly disturbed religious zealots who tormented the children, Rudyard in particular. The parents abandoned their children to complete strangers despite the fact that Mrs. Kipling had a large extended family in England. Neither child heard from their parents. Six years later, Rudyard's mother and father returned to England unannounced. Neither parent gave any apology for their extreme act of cruelty.

Rudyard called this dark, six-year period of his life the "House of Desolation." The severe psychological deprivation and abandonment led Rudyard to harbor strong unconscious feelings of hatred and bitterness toward his mother, which are reflected in many of his writings. Rudyard was saved from "soul murder" by the earliest loving years with his mother and father and by the activation of his prodigious creative gifts.

In his writings Rudyard both conceals and reveals his ambivalence and hatred of his mother for abandoning him. Echoes of Rudyard's intense rage and psychological pain come through in his poem "The Mother's Son," about a madman in a mental institution:

> I have a dream—a dreadful dream—
> A dream that is never done.
> I watch a man go out of his mind,
> And he is My Mother's Son...
> And it was *not* disease or crime
> Which got him landed there,
> But because They laid on My Mother's Son
> More than any man could bear...
>
> They broke his body and his mind
> And yet They made him live,
> And They asked more of My Mother's Son
> Than any man could give...

Kipling carried the emotional pain and burden of a mother and father who capriciously abandoned him. This wounding was particularly sharp-edged with regard to his mother. Much of this unconscious traumatic residue was transformed and manifested in his extraordinary gift of writing.

THE NATURE OF PSYCHOLOGICAL TRAUMA

Those who live in the aftermath of a relationship with a narcissist, whether it is a mother, father spouse or sibling, often experience psychological trauma. Psychological trauma is an attempt at the annihilation of the core self. Trauma can occur as one event or as a chronic condition of intolerable psychological pain that takes place over an extended period of time. The earlier in childhood the trauma occurs and the more chronic nature of the abuse, the greater the devastating emotional and psychological effects. With trauma, the child experiences a loss of personal security, is emotionally overwhelmed, feels unprotected and has pervasive feelings of helplessness. Trauma is psychologically tsunamic, a series of inescapable terror waves growing in power and height that carry the threat of death to the self.

How the Repetition Code is Set Up

The child of the narcissist suffers from varying levels of trauma from early childhood as a result of chronic exposure to a narcissistic parent. Being held at arm's length without affection or concern for his welfare, being treated as a worthless and inferior member of the family—these psychological blows are internalized into the child's psyche.

When we are small we are taught to believe that what our parents are communicating to us is true. We form much of our identity based on how we are treated by our parents and that affects what we believe about ourselves. Did the child feel genuinely loved and wanted? Did he feel neglected and dismissed? Did he feel threatened by the hatred of a parent toward him? Was he shamed, criticized and made to feel worthless? The answers to these questions affect the child's developing self-perception. Children of narcissistic parents often blame themselves; they look inside and feel inferior, ashamed, deficient and unwanted.

CRACKING THE CODE

Most people are unaware of their repetitive regressive behaviors, feelings and thinking patterns. When the consequences of narcissistic abuse become entrenched and self-destructive, the individual is trapped and unable to grow his gifts or sustain meaningful close relationships. Cracking the code of repetitive childhood and adult life narratives begins with the process of consciously identifying your psychological pain, expressing it and releasing it. Working through your core issues begins the evolution of the original true self—the spiral of growth, healing, individuation and transformation.

There is a center within us that is always seeking the truth about ourselves. Just as the body doesn't lie, neither does the infant. When the infant is frightened, surprised, angry or in physical pain, we observe him communicating his state of distress to us. We pick him up, soothe him, feed him and change him. Minutes after we put him down, the fussing and crying resumes. We observe more closely, checking all the clues that will tell us what is causing his distress. Many times we meet with success, sometimes by accident, and are able to resolve the baby's issue. He quiets and returns to a balanced emotional state.

Although infants are naturally able to communicate with us when they need something, as time goes on some children are forced to learn to conceal their real feelings. Narcissistic parents humiliate their children for displays of emotion. A narcissistic mother or father may openly laugh at a small child, telling him he is being silly or that he is a brat. The message is: "If you express how you are feeling, I will be very disappointed and angry with you. I expect a lot more of you. You must learn to control yourself or else." Expressing feelings signals emotional weakness to a narcissist, and many children of narcissists learn to keep their feelings inside, leaving them trapped in a repetitive cycle of non-expression.

Cracking the code of psychological repetition begins with waking up. When an individual is unaware of parental deprivations and childhood traumas they have suffered, these toxic remnants remain inside. When we are awake, we see things as they are, without delusion. There is no veil, wall or barrier that separates us from what is true. Trying to remain awake is a continuing battle. Some say it is a gift that we have come this far to be able to distinguish truth from delusion. Most people live in spiritual slumber. There are special souls we meet that give us the courage and wisdom to become more awake and follow our spiritual path.

Loosening the bonds of denial is our task and challenge. When we reject our true selves we are bound layer upon layer, ensnared by a Gordian knot that tightens with each denial of self. Recognizing and accepting blocked, psychologically injured parts of ourselves that have drifted from our unconscious minds is the next step in becoming an authentic individual. As children, we denied our feelings to survive. As adults who pursue the truth, we reclaim and express our feelings, own them and free ourselves from traumatic parental conditioning.

Identifying and releasing psychological wounds that drew emotional blood is essential to the evolution of our psyche and soul. Expanding the real self integrates us with our personal history and moves us forward as separate, individuated human beings.

SUMMARY OF THIS PROCESS

After cracking the code of the childhood survival repetition, successive awakenings form new psychological space. The old psychic structure loosens and the true self is consciously revealed, strengthened and manifested. As a result, the true self flowers with boundless gifts of imagination, creativity, empathy, intuition, compassion and joy. Hope is reborn, and with it the capacity to fulfill the dream and reality of the original authentic self.

The practice of stilling the mind (meditation in its many forms) creates a steadiness in the psyche that heals psychological and emotional wounds. It opens the heart to greater compassion, deepens intuition and drives creativity. This awakening is transpersonal, beyond our psychological life histories. Consistent practice of quieting the mind envelops us in a special calmness like the feeling of being gently held. Regular meditation strengthens the core of the psyche and opens the doors to higher consciousness.

Liberation is a process that is different for each individual. With liberation, the ego diminishes until it fades and disappears. We are at peace with the mortal wounds of childhood; we have mercy for ourselves and for others. Nature becomes a transcendent living entity where we find nourishment, inspiration and tranquility. The Eastern spiritual literature tells us that it is possible to reach liberation in this lifetime. Traveling this path, never to return, requires that we focus on wakefulness to the truth, clear discernment, loving-kindness, undaunted consistency, spiritual stamina and a rich rebounding sense of humor.

Checking Your Progress

- What are you doing to break the cycle of forming destructive relationships with narcissistic personalities? What strategies are working for you?

- Describe two core repetitions in your life.
- What have you learned about yourself as a result of your insights?
- How are you less psychologically and emotionally pulled toward narcissistic personalities?
- Name several ways you are becoming acquainted with your true self.

CHAPTER 4

Daily Writing Practice:
Discovering Unexpected Treasure

You should write, first of all, to please
yourself. You shouldn't care a damn about
anybody else at all … You have to live in such
a way that your writing emerges from it.

—DORIS LESSING

Actually, every time we begin, we
wonder how we did it before. Each time
is a new journey with no maps.

—NATALIE GOLDBERG

IF YOU HAVE LIVED WITH a narcissist, you have been constricted by that person's constant demands, criticisms
and humiliations for many years. Writing is one of the
best ways to free yourself from psychological oppression.

Growing up in a narcissistic family, we learn very early that we are not free to be our spontaneous selves. The narcissistic parent dictates and controls the life of his children. In some families, the narcissist observes that one or more of his offspring is handsome or beautiful, intellectually advanced, athletic, gifted in art or music or socially skilled. This dynamic operates in the child who is picked by the narcissist to be the "special golden one." This is the foundation for the creation of a false, grandiose self, a budding narcissist.

In other family constellations, the narcissistic parent takes an opposite role. They ignore and neglect their children. They cause deep psychological wounds, projecting their negative aggressive feelings, thoughts and impulses on to their children. Children targeted for abuse believe they deserve this abominable treatment. Many of them move through adulthood believing they are worthless, inadequate, weak, incompetent and bad human beings.

Both scenarios limit freedom of expression and require a healing process. As you heal in the aftermath of sharing your life with a narcissist, writing is one of the most powerful methods for loosening up, expressing your thoughts and emotions and igniting your imagination. Whether clothed in the art of fiction or spontaneously poured out without screening or editing, writing it is an act of freedom. Your writing, like your voice, DNA or fingerprint, is a unique expression of yourself. Writing transports you to surprising inner resources you may not have realized you had: receptivity to beauty, tenderness, insight and deep intuition, and direct access to the world of your unconscious.

All you have to do is open yourself up to writing. Without fear, shame or hesitation, write! No matter how you feel, what obligations you have, who is pressuring you, how much money you have or don't have, whether you are alone or surrounded by too many people, feeling emotionally vibrant, licking your wounds, feeling dejected or pissed off, write!

SPONTANEOUS WRITING

The practice of spontaneous writing is a gift that never wears out, has no restrictions or boundaries, and is always available. Writing is mysterious. You sit facing the computer screen or the white page and wonder how anything will appear. You might think, "My mind is blank," "My thoughts aren't flowing," "I feel shut down"—this is the inner critic that comes to sabotage you. Put the critic away for another time when he is needed. Be receptive to the natural vibration within you that is creating every moment. Hitch a ride on the flow and be carried by its force and momentum. It doesn't matter what you write, only that you sit and are receptive to what arrives from within.

Writing is un-choreographed. It rises from every layer of the unconscious. A seed of thought, a sliver of memory, a long-held regret, a secret beloved—they are all part of the mix. You are intrigued and fascinated. A skein of thread unwinds. The rhythm of the words picks up and you are dancing to its music. Become the instrument of this process. There are no speed bumps—no stopping to wonder if your spouse, mother, father, sister, brother will approve. Even if *you* don't approve, write it! Being a writer means never giving up on writing or your life.

Make a commitment to write each day. The amount of time that you spend writing is not as important as the consistency. You will be surprised, especially if you are open and nonjudgmental. At times writing becomes automatic. You are chasing the words, phrases and paragraphs faster than you can get them down.

Writing springs from the part of the mind that is free and expansive. Powerful feelings arise as we write in this way. They are connected with memories, longings, losses, pleasures, fantasies, traumas, terrors, guilt and fantasies. Writing hands you the absolute freedom to express anything that arrives.

Write, and make lots of mistakes. The voice you are hearing inside your head is urging you forward to run with its momentum. Write without shame, like a baby playing with his toes in the air. Shame has no place in writing. Doubt and fear have no entrance here. Whatever stops the natural flow of writing's river must remain on the shore.

When you write, go all out like the manic brush strokes in Van Gogh's paintings. Van Gogh's work looks wet. Your writing should feel like you've just been there, still warm from your fingertips. Write with the enchanting rhythms of Paul Simon, the velvet lilt of Ella Fitzgerald and the reflexive joy of Louis Armstrong.

WRITING AND PERSONAL TRANSFORMATION

Writing is a form of therapy that we carry with us and can use at any time. When we write we create people who never existed, bring the dead back to life and re-work our personal histories. Writing is a vehicle, it gives us a ticket to go as deep and far as we can imagine. We glimpse our soul's progress. We untie the painful knots of childhood, uproot what we couldn't bear to remember and spin entire worlds into existence.

Writing re-sets the default position of our life stories. It is one of the best activities you can perform as you heal from the pain and stress of life with a narcissistic spouse, parent, sibling or other family member. Writing transforms us. When we feel that we can no longer put one foot in front of another, we can write, feel the magic beneath our hands and in our heads and change our mood and life trajectory. Writing, we are re-born. Use writing to heal and transform yourself. Write in gratefulness. Write, knowing that there are no blocks. Write and know that you are never alone. Write what other people are afraid to say or think.

DIPPING INTO THE SPUN GOLD OF PROFESSIONAL WRITERS

We can learn so much about the writing process from professional writers, from their habits, routines and rituals. Professional writers use their personal life experiences in the most creative ways. Nothing goes by them.

Take Charlotte Armstrong, a gifted psychological suspense writer who wrote more than thirty highly acclaimed books, television dramas and two Broadway plays. Charl was a true intellectual—I learned more from her than in all of my formal years of schooling.

Charl was very disciplined. Her writing schedule began in the early morning. At noon she took a short break for lunch. Afternoons were devoted to re-writing and reading. She was fascinated by many diverse topics. When Charl became interested in a subject, she researched deeply and thoroughly.

Charl wrote seamlessly crafted plots and created characters from her rich imagination. She took her characters and stories from life, using composites of people she had known as well as developing characters as she wrote and letting them emerge through her creative alchemy. Charl was a master of dialogue. On many occasions her characters spoke spontaneously to one another and she wrote down their words. If she tried to change what they said, they insisted she leave it as originally spoken.

Charl was a voracious reader—three books a day in addition to her writing and intellectual studies, which included theology, philosophy, clinical psychology and literature. Charl kept dream journals for many years, analyzing her unconscious, developing a deep understanding of her own psyche. She was fascinated by diverse areas of knowledge, including the I Ching, the works of Shakespeare, Jungian psychology, mythology, theology and cosmology. Intellectual curiosity was one of Charl's greatest gifts. It was thrilling, sitting across from her, observing and feeling her extraordinary brilliance as our conversations on every topic imaginable traveled into the night.

For further inspiration for our daily writing practice, we can look to Irish writer William Trevor, who offers us a window into his personal creative process. Trevor is considered by many literary experts to be one of the greatest writers in the English language. He tells us: "I get melancholy if I don't [write]. I need the company of people who don't exist." Trevor explains that in order to be a writer one must be a social outsider, someone who can observe society from a distance. The great writer perceives the depths of human nature with its innumerable permutations and surprises.

Trevor describes himself as "an absolutely instinctive" writer: "To me, writing is entirely mysterious. If I didn't believe it was a mystery, the whole thing wouldn't be worthwhile." He doesn't plan his story endings nor is he concerned about endings during the writing process. He has faith that the next sentence will flow and arrive on the page. An example of the spun gold of Trevor's writing is from his novel, *The Story of Lucy Gault*:

> As the surface of the seashore rocks were pitted by the waves and gathered limpets that further disguised what lay beneath, so time made truth of what appeared to be ... The single sandal found among the rocks became a sodden image of death, and as the keening on the pier at Kilauran traditionally marked distress brought by the sea, so did silence at Lahardane.

What can we learn from observing the habits, practices and work of masterful professional writers? Besides the attributes of discipline, consistency and intellectual vigor, we appreciate the value of freeing up the unconscious mind and allowing it to speak its truth. Learning from every source—reading, listening, dreaming, life experiences—is the key to the creative quest. Creativity has neither limits nor boundaries; it is eternal, an endless horizon waiting for us to discover it.

WRITING AND OUR PERSONAL HISTORIES

Writing reveals what we have concealed and forgotten— the story we created in order to survive. When we write we go to the source, the truth about what happened to us: impossible dilemmas, moments of frozen terror, feelings of helplessness, being alone without anyone to take care of us and wondering if we could endure it. When we were little there was no escape. As we write now, we learn to revisit past experiences that were painful and intolerable. We feed them to ourselves in small doses that can be tasted, swallowed and digested by the practice and gift of writing. Although remaining fears still course through our bodies and minds, we can now sit with the pain, have mercy for the child inside who suffered and cradle her in our arms. Past life experiences emerge in every form: a memory faint or vivid, reoccurring fantasies, dreams that awaken us to the truth obfuscated by our intricately woven veils of delusion. Our personal histories fuel our creativity, and at the same time our creativity works to heal the deepest recesses of the psyche.

Great writers are mavericks; they don't fit into society. They tell the truth—that is not popular. No one wants to hear it: spouses, children, siblings, parents, friends and most others. This is because they cannot deal with the truth inside of themselves and are heavily shielded by their denial and delusion. When you tell the truth to most people, they first become afraid and then get angry with you because they cannot handle what they have hidden from themselves: secrets, psychological wounds, abandonments, painful cruelties and deprivations. All of this lurks in the dark storage of their unconscious and remains closed to those who cannot tolerate learning the core truths about themselves.

Those who are closed off to their core truths don't understand that writing lifts us beyond the pain of our personal histories. Using metaphor and imagination, we transform what has happened to us into an art form. We become anyone we wish. We use our own experiences as we write, but we also mold characters out of conscious and unconscious images and experiences we have never had.

Those who nourish the imagination and its enchantments are rewarded. Writing always surprises us; we cannot know beforehand what characters, landscapes, adventures or plots will appear in our minds. Becoming mentally and psychologically limber, receptive and non-judgmental are key factors in bringing these riches up to the surface and onto the page. We use all of our life experiences as well as the elixirs of our imaginations to invent the next character or story.

The greatest writers are living vessels of inspiration who not only work with the mysteries of the creative process; they surrender to them. Like these writers, we learn to embrace the mysterious. Communicating with the unconscious through spontaneous writing, we meet the evolving self, and to our surprise and delight discover there are neither limits nor rules, only the rhythm of the ecstatic flow.

WRITING AS A TRANSITIONAL OBJECT

Psychoanalyst D.W. Winnicott originated the term "transitional object," which he describes as a possession that a baby chooses as a source of comfort, usually a blanket, quilt or soft toy. At this time, the child is in a state of transition in his psychic development between being at one with mother and becoming psychologically separate from her. The transitional object plays the role of surrogate mother, representing the unconscious fantasy of the baby's bond with her. When the small child is alone or feeling the need to be close, he turns to the transitional object as a substitute mother. The chosen object is used to quiet rising separation anxiety and acts as a source of comfort that mitigates feelings of aloneness and restlessness and fear of abandonment. The transitional object is incorporated into the young child's rituals that provide him with needed soothing and calming.

As we look to recover from the psychological damage of the narcissist and heal ourselves, the act of writing serves as a transitional object and a psychological companion. We are the vessel of its creation, and it works to soothe us. When we write we may be physically alone, but as the process carries forward we are visited by memory traces, unconscious thoughts and vivid mental images. The writer feels the company of his own mind and the inhabitants of his imagination.

Different facets of our personalities arise as we write. Some are familiar, others foreign. These parts of the self have distinct voices. We turn a mental or emotional corner and find a fresh experience rising to greet us. As we open up, concealed fragments of our personalities come to life through our words. Activating the most innovative parts of the self takes place directly through engaging our intuition. This is writing's creative source. When we ride with intuition at our side and maintain a close relationship with it, we are directed by powerful forces that know and express truth.

Writing is a form of self-analysis, a process rather than a product, a flow without a reason, a wave that builds but doesn't need to reach shore. Writing is play, like jumping into the bluest sea on a summer day.

THE MUSIC OF WORDS

Writing is like spontaneous singing, allowing the voice to float on the notes it is discovering. Writing is a dance that we make up as we go along. We don't have to think about the steps; the body and mind know exactly where they want to go and how to get there. Writing is composing the music of words.

As a small child I grew up in a home where my grandfather arranged, composed and played music. Music was his essence as much as his beautiful open heart. I would watch him concentrating on a piece, quietly and quickly writing down notes, stops and pauses automatically as if some spirit were dictating to him. Once in a while he went to the piano and played a couple of chords, then returned to his music table to pursue his writing. My grandfather's concentration was powerful but relaxed, open but highly focused. The process of creating absorbed him and I knew he could hear every note of every instrument in his score. Hearing the music going through his mind, Papa was running like a river, waltzing through the rapids, moving into stiller waters— fused with the music that breathed through him.

Sometimes when Papa was free I would sing a melody, allowing the tune to flow out of me naturally. After I stopped, he repeated my melody on the piano and created an entire composition from it on the spot with exquisite harmonies and rhythms growing out of my original song. These experiences were very magical every time they happened and among the sweetest remembrances of my life.

I use this wonderful example to give you an idea of how words, like melodies, begin spontaneously, gather momentum, become intertwined and enlarged, ebb and flow and repeat their glorious song once again. As we make writing a daily practice, we become receptive to unborn words that are gestating deep inside of us.

CHECKING YOUR PROGRESS:

- How does your writing practice free up your creative juices?
- Name two of your favorite fiction writers. What touches you most about them and their work?

- How is the process of writing a source of companionship to you?
- What undiscovered parts of yourself have been revealed to you through your writing?

CHAPTER 5

Recovering through Your Creative Self

The Creative Artist and the poet and saint must
fight the actual gods of our society—the god
of conformism as well as the gods of apathy,
material success and exploitative power.

—ROLLO MAY

I dream of painting and then I paint my dream.

—VINCENT VAN GOGH

CREATIVITY IS OCCURRING EVERY MOMENT we are alive,
whether we are awake, asleep or dreaming or in joy,
sorrow or doubt. It is a transpersonal experience that
redeems us from our life histories. In the creative flow,
our identities are redefined. We jump into the roaring,

ecstatic stream, swept up in the current that created the cosmos and the tiniest infinitesimal cell.

Imagination is our creative engine. Like a sense of humor, imagination is unique to each person, our creative DNA. Having a rich imagination has advantages and disadvantages; it can carry us to ecstatic states or scare the hell out of us. Imagination dips deeply into the unconscious mind, the psyche where enchantment dwells. Unlike the finite, mundane world, imagination is infinite. Encourage the flow of your imagination. Be open—there are no rules, limits or boundaries. Follow where your imagination leads you.

DREAMS: CREATIVITY'S MESSENGERS

In slumber when the thinking mind is muted, we go into several sessions of REM (rapid eye movement) or dream sleep. This is a magical time, a creative oasis where the theater of the unconscious thrives. Carl Jung speaks eloquently about the nature of dreams: "The dream is a little hidden door in the innermost and most secret recesses of the psyche, opening into that cosmic night which was psyche long before there was any ego consciousness."

A friend mines his dreams as a source of creativity. He has what he calls "blockbusters," dreams that reveal in a highly dramatic and poetic form what he is feeling and thinking: his creative aspirations, repetitive cycles of behavior, conflicts, traumas and abandonments. These gifts of dreams come to him effortlessly, handing him the pure gold of the mystical unconscious.

Dreams are precious gems. They are our companions throughout life. They bring us inside the perpetual fires of creativity, alive with metaphors, images, sounds, words and colors that we take back with us to the waking world.

Exploring our dreams facilitates communication between our conscious and unconscious mind. These worlds become permeable and transparent to one another. Life is enriched by the surprising, often shocking, compressed images that well up automatically from the unconscious. Dream pictures are the mined gold of the psyche, the raw material of great art, the secrets to the real self and the mystical language that reunites us with the infinite.

THE SHADOW: GETTING TO KNOW YOU

Psychoanalyst Carl Gustav Jung introduced the archetype of the shadow, that part of the psyche that is largely unconscious and dispossessed. Jung observes: "The shadow personifies everything that the subject [person] refuses to acknowledge about himself" and represents "a tight passage, a narrow door, whose painful constriction no one is spared who goes down to the deep well." Those who have no conscious acquaintance with their shadow project forgotten, forbidden and disowned parts of themselves onto others in destructive ways.

The shadow not only contains the painful, sad, tragic elements of the psyche. Within the shadow are powerful, vibrant images of beauty, humor and truth. The shadow accesses precognitive messages, personal warnings and flashes of brilliance that come forth fully formed. Your shadow is as much a part of you as your breath. Without conscious acquaintance with our shadow, we are incomplete human beings. The creative notion of the shadow is not unique to psychoanalysis. The great painters da Vinci, Rembrandt, Raphael and Caravaggio used *chiaroscuro*, the Italian word for "light-dark," to build a rich contrast in their paintings, creating a dramatic solidity and multidimensional effect to their subjects. Their masterpieces possess qualities of depth, drama and aliveness.

Chiaroscuro used by the great painter Caravaggio in "Penitent Magdalene" presents us with the seated figure of Mary Magdalene. Her head, neck and shoulders are bowed in supplication. A small almost imperceptible tear runs down the side of her nose. Her full, white blouse, richly designed brown bodice and long skirt are in sharp contrast to the dark wall behind her. When we look at the painting, our eyes are drawn directly to the face of Magdalene and the profound eloquence of her posture of humility. There is a reaction that is both visceral and spiritual. We perceive her as an individual. We know her, feel her tragedy, anguish and resignation.

Our powerful response is due to the masterful use of chiaroscuro executed by Caravaggio. The light and dark blending makes his paintings both palpable and mysterious—they are living events.

Like the chiaroscuro that drew us into the "Penitent Magdalene," the interplay between light and dark is a humanizing force. Although we are not aware of it, we are confronted with light and dark in the psyche all of our lives. Most individuals have no conscious direct knowledge of their shadow. As a result, the shadow is expressed unconsciously through primitive verbal projections upon others and cruel deeds.

Your light cannot shine fully until your shadow is an integrated part of your essential self. Once you embrace your shadow it releases unbounded sources of creativity into the psyche. We are made of light and dark, like every living entity; integrate your shadow, learn its language, welcome its messages, and be thankful you have found one another.

The integrated shadow adds a lively juiciness to the individual personality. There is a marked difference between this person and those who have their shadows tightly hidden in the unconscious. When we are receptive to our shadow and invite it in, we notice its distinctive, multicolored presence in our dreams, fantasies, conversations, writings and reveries. The shadow does not reveal itself to us completely; many of its workings remain a mystery. As we become receptive and open to our shadow we receive unexpected gifts in the form of creative inspirations, aesthetic visions and wisdom about our true nature.

When kept out of conscious awareness, the shadow overruns the personality. Like the shadow of the moon in midday eclipses the sun, everything becomes dark. The disowned shadow takes retribution against the closed personality, revealing itself in highly destructive ways. Those who have no conscious acquaintance with their shadow project psychologically disavowed parts of themselves onto others. The shadow elements that control an individual's personality are a lethal poison that affects those closest to him—spouses, children and siblings.

Obstructing the shadow also leads to a lack of precious spontaneity, a dampening of emotional expression and the incapacity to be fully alive. People constrained by fanatical religious orthodoxy are chained to their unconscious shadow like an albatross that pulls them down into the deepest sea bottom.

One way or another the shadow seeps out, rushing from its hiding place and flooding the personality. The individual who is this tightly wound loses control over his unconscious and seriously disrupts and upends the lives of others.

Incorporating the shadow into the conscious personality and welcoming the richness of this unconscious archetype plays a major role in individuation and the unfolding of the true self. The shadow is a conundrum. We can visualize contacting our shadow as a series of dance moves. When we learn to dance, first we concentrate on each step and body position. We practice these sequences many times. Gradually, with a lot of consistent work, the routine feels natural. At some point the steps, rhythm and body movements become synchronized.

One of the most accessible ways to dance with your shadow is through your daily writing practice. As you become familiar with spontaneous writing you find yourself moving with the tide, the words coming in torrents, pouring through your mind and imagination. You will be surprised at the endless images and scenes presented to you by your shadow. You think: "How is this possible? This is not me." Gradually you recognize and accept that you are filled with rich material that has remained unfamiliar until now.

The pure brilliance and imaginative power of the shadow cannot be overestimated. All great art—painting, sculpture, dramas, comedies, dance, literature, etc.—embraces elements of the shadow that burst with freshness, eloquence, spontaneity and mystery.

Dreams are filled with newly born shadow images. In dreams we experience what is impossible in waking life. Creatures, human and inhuman, make their appearance on our nightly stage. We are fascinated, appalled, terrified, engaged and in awe of them. Where did they come from? What force inside of us created them? They are earthly and otherworldly, heavenly and demonic.

You can be anyone or anything when working with your shadow. You play every role: low down, high born, Queen, King, athlete, dancer, saint, criminal, survivor, victim, soldier, ninja, painter, prehistoric man. You wander with the snow leopards of the Himalayas, you ride on the back of a mother whale in the Sea of Cortez, you raise your head to the chilling winds and howl with the Siberian wolves.

INTUITIVE SIGHT

Intuitions are moments of insight that awaken our consciousness with warp speed and clarity. I hear people ignoring or overriding their intuition. These messages can appear to be irrational or too novel for those who are strongly influenced by the analytical mind. In today's societal milieu, which is oriented outward toward action, material acquisition and blind ambition, the voice of intuition is not valued and becomes muted.

Attaining and using this kind of truth communicated to us is rare in Western society. When you are an intuitive, many people label you as an eccentric or as psychologically unbalanced. This can be hard, but at some point in our lives it is vital to cast aside how others perceive us. You may have fewer friends when you live and communicate from your inner core self, but these friendships are authentic and invaluable.

Psychological openness is key to deepening intuition. The intuitive message is faster than thought. With intuition, one doesn't ponder. Remaining flexible and still invites intuition. Growing up in a family that values these perceptions is a benefit, but developing and refining intuition can be achieved at any stage of life.

HUMAN TRAGEDY AND CREATIVITY

Some individuals live through tragedy—early loss of a parent, physical and psychological abuse, maternal deprivation. Tragedy places an imprint on the psyche. Individuals who experience tragedy are different from those whose lives have been uninterrupted by this level of severe psychological and emotional pain.

We are molded by the pain and sorrow we have suffered and endured. Many who experience tragedy and trauma blot it out through repression, which is an unconscious defense mechanism that leads to a "forgetting," as if these events never occurred. Others turn to their intellect to protect themselves from their feelings and become psychologically numb. This strategy saves them from psychological pain but robs them of access to the full expression of feelings and emotions.

Some people lead smooth lives. They focus on the externals—their possessions, outward appearance and image, how they are viewed by others, their social milieu and the power of their professional status.

These individuals lack an understanding of their inner selves and are oblivious and disinterested in living authentically.

I have observed that those who always sail on life's unruffled seas have deep psychological, emotional and empathic characterological gaps. They are unfamiliar with their core selves. They are incurious and resistant to comprehending tragedy, sorrow, loss, despair or psychological pain. If you speak about these matters, they accuse you have being negative and self- absorbed. Others whisk themselves away, making excuses and hasty exits. The doors you attempt to open, they keep locked and sealed. You have gotten too close to their unconscious core of childhood traumas and deprivations. They fear you are going to discover the dreaded key to what is concealed inside of them. This avoidance, the putting up of impenetrable barriers, speaks loudly of the truth about themselves and their family histories.

If tragedy is a core part of your personal history, make use of it. Tragedy transforms and deepens those who deal with it consciously. It leads to a search for the soul. When everything has been stripped away, there is nowhere to go but the center, the origin. When consciously processed and worked through, tragedy leads us through delusion to truth.

Like tragedy, suffering, when acknowledged, understood and released, creates new neuronal and spiritual pathways. It enriches and deepens the metaphors of your life, the territories of your imagination and the thematic narrative of your dreams.

From life's suffering, lasting beauty can be created. Rembrandt van Rijn's masterpieces are a testament to a life filled with tragedy. Rembrandt's life was one of highest artistic achievement and innovation combined with a personal history of great tragedy. Rembrandt's creative genius was obvious from his early years. At the beginning of his career, Rembrandt was financially successful, selling his paintings and acquiring many commissions. By his mid-thirties he had endured the loss of his wife Saskia (age 30) and three of his children. He lived too lavishly, fell heavily into debt and eventually became bankrupt.

Despite a series of tragedies, Rembrandt's extraordinary artistry deepened and his works became more profound. Tragic fate pursued him in later life. His common law wife Hendrickje died at the age of twenty-seven followed by the death of his son Titus.

Rembrandt left us with an unsurpassed artistic legacy against the backdrop of a difficult life filled with personal pain and loss. His presence is felt in every work, his humanity on every canvas and his greatness in every stroke. In Rembrandt's eyes and expression we feel a deep sense of knowing; he carries the full burden of being human. In his self-portraits, Rembrandt is psychologically transparent. There is no veil, no façade and no barrier. He invites us to look deeply inside and to know the full truth of our being.

NATURE AND CREATIVITY

When we enter the natural world, everywhere we turn we experience billions of shapes, colors, hues and rhythms. Nature is ever changing, persistently at work creating new life forms.

Nature stretches the imagination and enriches us in a very personal way. Nature's canvas pulsates with life and death—a terrible beauty. The infinite varieties of evolving life found in nature teach us to approach our days as adventurers and seekers.

We are part of this creation that throbs at the center of our being. We were meant to live surrounded by nature's abundance. The great Renaissance painter Leonardo Da Vinci, who spent much of his life outdoors, gives voice to nature's indispensability: "Human subtlety will never devise an invention more beautiful, more simple or more direct than does nature because in her inventions nothing is lacking, and nothing is superfluous."

Nature provides us with innumerable gifts of beauty and creativity. The bird's nest is ingenious in its variety and intricacy of design and choice of materials and locations. Each bird species produces a distinct nest that protects eggs and baby birds from the elements and predators. Nests are built in ground tunnels, tree holes, on water and high in the tallest forests. From the grand aerie of the eagle to the tiniest cup-shaped refuge of the thimble-sized hummingbird, these designs defy our imagination.

Nature announces that beauty is never-ending, that each leaf is an individual, that every mother seal recognizes the special sound of her baby's call, that mother elephants protect and care for their small calves with graceful tenderness.

Creativity and nature are close companions. An artist friend gardens when she is not painting. She experiences great joy planting trees, flowers, shrubs and bushes to create a living work of art for each season. Her garden and her paintings intertwine with one another in a constant process of re-creation. Her attunement with nature, fearlessness in trying new techniques and sense of wonder and openness are an integral part of her paintings.

All creativity begins with nature, and even the greatest artists cannot replicate her beauty, eternal variety, paradoxes and mysteries—she confounds and seduces us. Watching several films of the Great Barrier Reef, I entered a world that was so magnificent that it was difficult to believe it was real. From space, the Great Barrier Reef is called the Blue Opal, an expanse of sea over 2,000 kilometers long. As you enter its waters you are surrounded by the vibrant color, shape, design, pulse and rhythm of every living sea creature imaginable. The reef is made up of the skeletons of sea animals, which have created its growing foundation, textures and shapes over the last 15,000 years. It is roiling with dynamic, ever-changing patterns of design, color, shape and form that depend on the water's movements— countless schools of fish, hundreds of varieties of corals, leviathans of the sea like the whale shark and the giant eel.

This pulsating beauty of infinite variety takes us out of our everyday minds and lifts our consciousness. Our personal doors of perception open more fully. We are receptive to ever-expanding possibilities for creating a new life that moves toward wholeness and thrives on beauty. Each creature in this mystical place is unique, yet all are interdependent for food, cleaning, protection, procreation and camouflage. When we take in the immense glory of natural wonders like the Great Barrier Reef, we are freed up to experience our inner and outer worlds in penetrating depth.

ARTISTS OF THE PALEOLITHIC—OUR BROTHERS

A week before Christmas in 1994, three spelunkers were exploring the limestone cliffs of Pont d'Arc in south-central France. As they moved across a natural bridge of rock, they felt cold air coming from an updraft on the cliff's ledge, which hinted that there might be an open cavity, a cave. Eliette Brunel, the physically slightest of the climbers, squeezed herself through a thin passage. The others followed, leading them to a magnificent cathedral-like space filled with exquisite Paleolithic art. Eliette Brunel cried: "They have been here!" She was looking at the phenomenal paintings displayed throughout a vast series of rooms within interconnecting caves. Until this moment no human being had seen this collection of art masterpieces for over 30,000 years. Using the undulations and textures of the caves' surfaces, the artists had produced three-dimensional-like paintings. In the different galleries there was a variety of beautifully executed colored and charcoal drawings of Stone Age animals: rhinos, lions, bison and a magnificent frieze of horses and ibex. Artists had gathered and worked in the caves for thousands of years to paint their surroundings, especially the animals with whom they shared their lives. On the far side of some caves, individual artists had pressed their red-pigmented palms against the wall, leaving their signature.

The discovery of those theatres of caves, archways and pavilions containing the finest Stone Age art ever discovered inspires us to remember who these people were and who we are. In a flash, 30,000 years of time vanishes. We are one with our ancestors, pressing our palms on theirs as we enter the ecstatic, creative flow of life and art.

Trios of horses, sublimely drawn and painted, arrest our gaze. Deer and bison are rendered with great detail by artists who lived with these animals daily. Within the

Chauvet Cave are glorious paintings of hundreds of animal species that had never been discovered: bears, lions, panthers, hyenas and rhinoceroses. In this great Paleolithic cathedral we make close contact with the artists who speak to us through the masterpieces they have left— the Chauvet Caves reminds us of our shared creativity and humanity with our Paleolithic brothers.

GLORIOUS COLOR

Color saturates our reality. It follows us everywhere like a chorus of angels. We see color awake and asleep, when we are sick or well, in love or out, in mania or depression. Without color, life lacks vibrancy. Some individuals experience color more vividly than others, not because of the condition of their eyesight but because of the receptivity of their psyches.

Color speaks to each person with a different voice. We remember colors with fondness, nostalgia, romance, loss or affection. One example of the emotional power of color is the deep rose-red velvet couch of my early childhood. It was removed without my knowing. It disappeared; no explanation was given. There was something special about that couch that had meaning for me: the touch of the velvet against my body when I sat on it, the regal color that had become a part of my everyday life. For me, the velvet couch represented a kind of consistency I could rely upon. When it was gone, part of my security evaporated. The couch was not treasured because it was expensive or opulent, but due to the memories it held for me. It was the smooth texture, inviting shape, and deep, mysterious rose-red that filled me with an experience of familiar, cozy beauty.

Color is our life companion, telling us "Everything is alive!" Communicating directly with color, we are immersed and saturated by it vividness. We put our emotional pain in the background when color vibrates before our eyes and fills all our senses. Color is full of surprises, taking us on journeys of the imagination.

THE CREATIVE POWER OF THE SENSE OF PLACE

For millennia artists have used a sense of place to shape and deepen their creativity. The impressionist painter, Claude Monet, envisioned, and built with exquisite detail, his estate and gardens at Giverny, on the right bank of the River Seine. Monet purchased land that had been inhabited since Neolithic times, designed his house and gardens and worked into creation every shape, color, texture, flower and plant that he would paint by hand. Monet's profound sense of place inspired his great masterpieces: "Gardening was something I learned in my youth ... I perhaps owe having become a painter to flowers."

What is your sense of place? Is it located in the memories of your childhood, a product of your imagination, scenes that inhabit your dreams and fantasies? Our sense of place can be made out of any experience. It can be a compilation of memory fragments from trips we have made decades ago. Reaching back, we evoke the colors, sounds, aromas, tactile sensations and tastes of these events long held and sweetened by the imagination. Your travels, near or far, concrete or imagined, remain with you, ever-present for recollection and re-living. Finding your sense of place solidifies psychological grounding and promotes emotional security.

RIDING MUSIC'S WAVES

Those who grow up with music are doubly blessed. Music resounds through the body and mind, awakening and expanding our human possibilities. Music takes us away from distracting conscious thoughts and into a sensory world of relaxation and freedom. Music urges our bodies to move, sway, swing and glide. It enlivens our torsos and limbs to respond to the story it is telling. Music shifts our moods when they are gray, or even black, or balance on fear's razor edge. We feel music pulsate through our bodies from the ground to our splayed feet, winding through every chakra and shooting out through the tops of our heads. When we ride on music's waves, we are caught like a surfer in the ecstatic tube of the curl. Music is eternal—its rhythms, melodies and grace notes pulse through our blood and breath, lifting us to ascension.

Music transports us to other worlds. Our attitudes shift, our spirits lighten; we shed our emotional burdens. Music encompasses our whole body, mind, senses and emotions. Immersing in music, becoming a part of it and fusing with its magic opens up our spontaneity. Going through the veils of external reality into the music, we let go of our personal histories. With every note and sequence, we move deeper into music's rich world of mystery and beauty. We are carried along, we float, we rise with music's waves. Great music surprises and calms us. It is a friend that soothes us, lifting our heavy hearts and smoothing out the deep wrinkles of our disillusionments. Music dilutes our fears. We wonder where they have gone, but before we can answer the melody resumes and carries us on its unchartered winds to a new adventure.

The miracle of melody causes us to cry, touches the mortally wounded heart and opens it with notes from heaven. Melodies fill the gaps in our inner baby's longings and heal the scars of hatred and terror we have borne. Melodies are eternal.

A friend of mine had a peak experience on her first trip to New Orleans. She and a group of friends entered Preservation Hall, a historic location in the French Quarter devoted to jazz. Vanessa described her response to the special music that filled her being: "I became entranced with the sounds and syncopations of the jazz group. As they wound up I became ecstatic, feeling an intense vibration move throughout my body from the bottom of my feet through my spinal column and out through the crown of my head. It was transcendent joy."

Music creates a different sense of space inside ourselves. We glide along its whirls, rhythms and enchanting melodies. Music draws us into its magic. We cannot resist it. When we learn to appreciate it, music becomes part of our heartbeat and the rhythm of our breath. Fine music, whether classical or popular, imprints enduring pictures in our minds. It heals what we cannot forget and smooths the sharp edges of our psychological pain. Music lyrics lead us on a journey where we are happily lost, following a mesmerizing ribbon of words.

Creativity is dynamic. Day and night you are invited to slip into the creative stream running by and within you. As you touch your aliveness and freedom, creativity's ecstatic flow embraces you. Ride it like the Andean condor god of the sky, circling in wide arcs hour after hour, winging effortlessly on thermals thousands of feet above the earth.

CHECKING YOUR PROGRESS:

- Describe three themes from your dreams. What are the deepest insights you have had from dreams?
- How are you becoming acquainted with your shadow?

- How has trauma or tragedy fueled your creativity?
- Describe two peak life experiences you have had in nature.
- What are your favorite colors? Why do you love them so much? How do they make you feel?
- Describe the place of music in your life. How does it lift your spirits, calm you down, let the tears flow, act as your intimate companion?

CHAPTER 6

Friendships: Trust and Transformation

The job of a friend is not to decide what
should be done, not to run interference or
pick up the slack. The job of a friend is to
understand, and to supply energy and hope ...

—MERLE SHAIN

...True friendship is a kind of singing.

—THOMAS MERTON

WITH A FRIEND, WE TAKE a journey. The closer friends
become, the deeper they are able to touch the core of
one another and themselves. Close friends reach under-
standings, express emotions, and tell long-held secrets.
A friend helps us ride out our regressive emotional states
when we rant, cry, complain or howl into the crosswinds

of our distress. Friends are steady when we feel thrown and confused. They help us to bear what is unbearable and deal with what almost crushed us.

BEING HEARD

True friendships provide us with an environment to be heard on every level. Friends are receptive to our periods of regression and growth, our seasons of sorrow and joy.

Fostering a true friendship can be especially difficult for those who have grown up with narcissistic parents or been married to a narcissist. If you've had a relationship with a narcissist, you may have been restrained and controlled from expressing yourself and exposed to perpetual criticism. Showing your feelings or expecting to be treated kindly when you are emotionally vulnerable is met with disgust. You cannot have an authentic relationship with or place trust in these individuals; they will always betray you. Living with a narcissist as a child or spouse places you in the role of serving them and keeping their egos fully inflated.

Developing a true friendship can help us recover from these damaging experiences. We begin to share ourselves in ways we have never ventured with another human being. With a true friend, hope and trust are strengthened and renewed.

When we share the intimacy of a genuine friendship we are never alone, whether that person is physically present or not. We carry their image, voice, words, and gestures within us.

Friends take on different roles. We are playmates having fun, being silly. The trusted friend is a protector, like a loving parent. A friend helps us ride out our painful emotional states when we feel overwhelmed. Crying in front of a friend is comforting; there is no shame or awkwardness. We feel at home within ourselves as we express our raw feelings.

PSYCHOLOGICAL CONTAINER

A friend is a psychological container of our life history—everything about us is held in that person's heart. Like part of our DNA, there is an intrinsic need to find others who can hold and contain our deepest feelings when we cannot bear them. This person is available when we need them, not when it is convenient. A friend stays with us regardless of time. The true friend makes the extra effort to comfort us, to hold us psychologically. We can reveal our secrets and inner darkness to them and not be judged.

In utero the mother is the physiological container that provides the embryo with total sustenance. After birth the infant is held in the mother's arms, fed, caressed and taken care of completely. As the baby grows, he is able to move more freely, laugh, gesticulate, concentrate and express different emotions. With all of these developmental accomplishments, mother maintains the role of psychological container to her baby. As the child becomes more independent, he still turns to mother to tend to his needs, to be listened to and understood, to have his emotions deciphered and contained when he is overwhelmed and out of control. Gradually, through the years, the child internalizes these repeated ministrations of the mother and becomes capable of feeling secure out of mother's presence and coping with challenges and frustrations that arise.

No matter how mature we are, human beings have a need to be understood. We search to find true friends who can hold and contain our deepest feelings. We carry them inside when we are lonely, weary and devastated. They listen with kindness and never give up on our progress through difficult and painful life passages.

FRIENDSHIPS INSPIRE CREATIVITY

When we are respected and understood, we feel free to share our dreams and creative ideas. With friends, ideas swirl, thinking coalesces and insights stir. We share our inspirations openly. Friends are generous with their ideas and give them away to us when we are uninspired or need their collaboration on a personal problem or creative challenge.

Friends widen our personal and professional horizons. We are more able to take chances in using our creative gifts and making leaps that would be much more difficult if we were alone. We know that if our projects fail in the world, if our efforts go unrewarded, if we are treated with unjustifiable cruelty, our friend will always be present to empathize with our painful experiences and to help restore our psychological equilibrium.

Close friends are more than the sum of two. Their devotion, comfort, loyalty, creative solutions—everything they bring from their lives—increases our feelings of abundance and hope. True friends have respect for one another's personal boundaries but are so trusted that they go very deep into each other's psyches

When you are speaking with a good friend, an easy flow takes place. If you are working on a creative project, you are free to allow ideas to tumble out of your mind spontaneously, with no hesitation or embarrassment. Listening intently, your friend gives clear feedback and offers new ideas and ways of achieving your goal. Friends want you to succeed and they will do everything they can to propel you forward. A close friend is an inspiration, especially at those times when you feel you have run dry or are too psychologically jagged or worn out to come up with fresh ideas.

Friends are always thinking about you. You are an integral part of their psyche; sometimes they know you better than you know yourself. A good friend can be halfway across the world but be intimately present for you. Some friends have intuitive perceptions between one another; a way of communicating that is beyond words.

A good friend will drop his schedule to see you through a crisis. There are no limits to the times that you can ask for support, ideas, understanding and empathy. Like a mother who is keenly aware of her child throughout the days and nights of his life, the great friend is always there.

TELLING US THE TRUTH

Friends stand in our blind spots and tell us the truth about ourselves when we are too deluded to see it. They confront us in a compassionate way. Their view is uncluttered by the ingrained psychological history we carry. They know our personal history, and because of this can detect better than we can where our view is obstructed. At times when we may see through a glass darkly, their vision is clear and accurate.

Friends are protective of our welfare, even to the finest detail. They instinctively know when we need solitude to sort out our thoughts and feelings. Close friends are keepers of our secrets. Everyone has secrets—there are secrets we tell a few friends, secrets we share with those closest to us and secrets that stay with us forever. To know someone intimately, you have to know his or her secrets. A secret is often the missing piece that solves the puzzle of the self. Secrets conceal themselves in the caverns of the unconscious. Secrets unremembered can become life patterns that are repetitive and self-destructive.

FRIENDS GO THE DISTANCE

Marathon runners talk about an excruciating experience some of them have after the twenty-mile mark of the race called the wall, which occurs as a result of glycogen depletion in the muscles. There is a feeling of complete enervation in the body, needing to stop, knowing you cannot take another step. At this point the body and mind are screaming at the runner to drop out of the race, but they keep going. Much of their perseverance is based on their disciplined years of training, their unequivocal devotion. There is something mystical about the great distance runner. In the midst of the wall, despite all his physical symptoms and the pull of his emotions, he can visualize the finish line. He will keep going; there is no other alternative for him.

This metaphor applies to great friendships. Friends outlast the twists and turns of one another's lives, the tragedies that are weathered, the down periods when marital relationships are rocky, the illness that afflicts one or both of them or their families. We hit our walls—betrayals, depression, addictions, panics, and economic upheavals and don't think we can tolerate it for another moment. Then we call up our friend and he or she comes and moves us through the wall, helping us regain sight of the finish line.

FRIENDSHIPS SUPPORT PSYCHOLOGICAL AND SPIRITUAL GROWTH

In many ways, good friends act as informal therapists to one another. Mutual empathy is a source of healing to both parties. In some cases a friend is as effective at helping us heal as a professional psychotherapist.

Friends encourage our spiritual growth through their devotion and love. A person doesn't have to belong to a formal church to be spiritual. Spirituality is highly personal, it is defined by what resonates deeply within us and leads us to the higher consciousness of loving kindness, mental spaciousness, deep intuition and actions that alleviate the suffering of others. A friend respects how you define your spiritual life, and his or her support helps you grow.

You are a witness to the changes your friend makes within himself, the personal battles he wins and those he loses. The gentleness of having a friend reminds us that we have to work on our sharp edges, to mute our judgmental tone and to give others a break even when we envy them.

When a friend dies, we feel the wrenching pain that only they can evoke in us. We are left with their essence and the experiences we had with them. The rich histories we have written together resonate within our souls.

Many years ago, I became friends with an extraordinary woman named Shannon. She was such an individual, with boundless energy and joie d' vivre. She and I would stand in the middle of our yards and laugh so loudly we would almost burst. At times, the contagion of our laughter disrupted the quiet of our uptight neighborhoods. I tried to keep it down for the neighbors, but it was impossible when she and I got into the groove. Even now, I can hear her laugh as I am writing.

Shannon led a very difficult life because of her health and her family. She was diagnosed with diabetes at the age of seven. Shannon's mother was a critical, demanding woman who tried to control her at every turn—she spent much of her life trying to please this impossible woman. Fortunately, she had a loving father who cared deeply about her.

One very significant event in Shannon's life was a near-death experience, which occurred when she was eighteen. She had gone into a diabetic coma, and remembered herself in the hospital drifting away. She described the beautiful colors surrounding her: aquamarines, sea foam greens, vivid rose-pinks, violets, amethysts, brilliant golds. Shannon rose up to the ceiling and watched as her parents huddled together and the doctors and nurses worked on her to save her life. Near the end of the experience, she descended from her high perch, and as she floated down the colors and aromas of flowers filled her senses. She heard a voice say, "She's back now," and realized she had returned to her body. She cherished this near-death experience and appreciated its revelations and loveliness. She described it as one of the most beautiful events of her life.

Throughout our friendship, Shannon watched out for me. I was in her mind. She surprised me with little cards and small gifts at unexpected times. When I told her how much I loved butterflies, she gave me a tiny book about finding the right flowers to grow in my garden to attract them.

She loved cooking special meals and baking. She loved animals, and frequently fed the blue jays in her yard, peanut by peanut, from the palm of her hand. She was a master storyteller. She often got carried away with silliness, and I went right along with her for a fantastic ride!

As she grew older, the burden of her childhood illness became greater and she faltered physically. She moved, and I missed her. She sent me lovely cards of animals and plants and flowers. One day I found out that she had been hospitalized and was near death. I visited her and felt the deep wound of losing her—though she was technically alive, the Shannon I had known was no longer present. After a short time, she left the body. I have never stopped thinking about her and loving her. Her voice and stories come into my mind often.

CHECKING YOUR PROGRESS:

- What personal and characterological qualities do you look for in a close friend?
- Name several ways your friends have inspired your creativity.
- How did a friend help you get through a very difficult time?
- Tell a short story about a wonderful friend.
- How do friends support your psychological and spiritual growth?

CHAPTER 7

Meditation: Healing through Inner Stillness

Every time we become aware of a thought,
as opposed to being lost in a thought, we
experience that opening of the mind.

—JOSEPH GOLDSTEIN

While absorbed in meditation ... it is imperative
to remain wide awake ... What is the outcome
of such meditation? It opens up one's being
to the light, to that which is eternal.

—SRI ANANDAMAYI MA

MEDITATION IS THE KEY TO insight, healing, and breaking unproductive and distructive patterns of behavior. It calms the mind, opens the heart and awakens the soul. Meditation takes us beyond the recycling chatter of crowded thoughts. With meditation, we reach the mind beyond mind, thought beyond thought—the source of knowing. In deep meditation we experience a vibration of peace.

If you have shared your life with a narcissist, whether a parent, spouse, sibling, you have been constantly bombarded by their demands, intimidations and cruelties. Manipulated and exploited, you have waited in a state of apprehension and dread for the next assault. When you live with a narcissist, nothing is private or sacred. The space in which you move is not your own; the narcissist's restlessness and rage permeate the household. Even when there is physical distance, you feel their overwhelming presence. They crowd your mind and block your internal space. Meditation allows you to free yourself from the bonds of the narcissist and regain your mental space.

Each meditation is unique. As we sit, it is normal for our minds to swing and jump from thought to thought, feeling to feeling, sensation to sensation, like gusts of wind. We meander through worn ruts of life experiences, fragments of dreams, old fears, gnawing guilt, lingering regrets.

Working consistently with your meditation practice, you incrementally strengthen your ability to focus and remain open. Cultivating the quality of being open and present without the inner critic is essential to your practice. As you begin to meditate, many thoughts appear. This is a signal that you are aware of your inner process. Your meditation practice has begun.

Accept each sitting with an open mind. Feelings come up to the surface and demand attention. You find yourself in a maze of repetitious thinking and etched memories. The urge to stop is tempting. Gently acknowledge to yourself that you are all right just where you are. If your mind, senses and feelings were not swirling, you would not be meditating. As your practice becomes consistent, you will notice that there are quieter times inside. Give yourself credit every time you sit and make the effort. This the most important act of all.

Go to your place of meditation each day despite how you feel psychologically or emotionally about it. If you wait until you "feel" like meditating, it is not going to happen. I know a few meditators who can't wait to sit, but these people are rare. Don't compare yourself with anyone else. If you have been meditating for years, you find there are periods of time or individual sessions in which you are distracted by obsessive thoughts, impulses, physical discomfort and emotional irritations. In the midst of these intermissions and interruptions, you are still meditating.

Don't let others make judgments about your meditation process. This is between you and the higher consciousness within you. Don't label a meditation as good or bad. Spiritual movement is not measured in days, weeks or years. Meditation is an organic process; it has its own pace and remains mysterious.

Consistent meditation practice has profound health-enhancing effects on the body. It reduces stress by regulating cortisol levels, lowering blood sugar, strengthening the immune system and increasing the quality of brain functioning.

Meditation creates a spaciousness of mind. When we are at peace, even for a few moments, we expand and deepen. The ego, the "me" voice that speaks the language of self-importance and extreme self-entitlement, is muted. Our personal life history, with all of its psychological burdens and wounds, recedes. We touch the source of inner peace.

CHANTING: RAISING THE VOICE IN DEVOTION

Chanting is natural to the human voice. When we chant, we loosen the bonds of entrenched thought patterns. We feel the pull of a calming, wordless inner world. Chanting carries us to new vibrations where we discard the burden of our psychological defenses and personal histories. When we chant, we express in sound the calls of our human and animal ancestors: the wolf's midnight howl, the nightingale's warble, the rook's caw, the fox's yip.

In 1967 the French physician, psychologist and ear specialist Alfred Tomatis studied the beneficial effects of the performance of Gregorian chants on a group of Benedictine monks. For hundreds of years, it was the practice of the monks to chant six to eight hours a day with a few hours of sleep. This disciplined schedule worked for them, but a new director of the abbey omitted this practice. After their chanting practice had stopped, the monks reported that they felt very fatigued and had difficulty sleeping. In studying the monks' physical complaints, Dr. Tomatis came to the conclusion that chanting energized their brains and bodies. Dr. Tomatis explained that the monks "had been chanting in order to 'charge' themselves."

The chanting of *Om* has been intoned for thousands of years in the Indian culture and elsewhere in the world. *Om* is a Sanskrit word that means *avati* or *rakuati,* "One who protects, sustains." So that which sustains everything is *Om. Om* is the original vibration that was intoned before the universe came into existence.

Chanting calms the nervous system, slows and deepens the breathing rate, quiets the heart and lowers the blood pressure. When we chant, we shift from the sympathetic nervous system of the survival fight-or-flight syndrome to the parasympathetic nervous system of calmness and healing. You can create your own chants by experimenting with different sounds you produce. It is a relaxing experience, knowing that you don't have to think, follow directions or obey anyone else's rules. Be free and open with your sounds. Have fun with them.

MAKING THE EFFORT

Two vital actions to your meditation practice are making the effort and being consistent. If you sit for two minutes, even one minute each day, you will make more progress than if you were meditating for an hour once a week. Meditation accumulates like a force of nature. It is a ritual that eventually becomes a habit. Even when your meditations feel unsteady and strewn with random thoughts and distracting body sensations, you are meditating. Do not judge the quality of your meditation. Trust the process as it works through you.

Don't think about how others have described their flights into *Samadhi*, the astral sounds that float into their ears or the elaborate visions they behold. Don't be distracted by the hours that devotees spend prostrate and unmoving on their perches. That is their experience, or more accurately, that is what they are telling you about it. This is your meditation, your effort, your process.

MEDITATION IS PERSONAL

Meditation is not one-size-fits-all. Create a specific place in your home that you use for meditation. You may want to put pictures, icons, small smooth stones or candles there to remind you of your meditation practice. Wear comfortable clothing. Try to meditate around the same time each day if it's possible. When you meditate, make it as comfortable and pleasant as you can.

Consistency in meditation is key, but don't punish yourself when you miss a meditation. Even if it is weeks or months, return to your practice. You are a meditation prodigal who has come back to seek the peace and insight you need, deserve and are destined to have. Be grateful, have no regrets. You have come back home.

There are experiments of Tibetan Buddhist monks who wrapped themselves in water soaked sheets and sat outside in freezing weather. Within a short time, the monks were wearing warm dry sheets that had been transformed in temperature and texture through the changes in body temperatures during deep meditation. For our purposes, drying wet sheets worn in bone-chilling snow is not the goal. Do not seek perfection in meditation. If your thoughts are running and jumping about, let that be. If your emotions are on high and ripping you away from concentration on your breath, that's ok. Make peace with your attitude toward yourself. When you sense negativity and self-reproach creeping into your thoughts, acknowledge this like watching a leaf floating on a river. Let it move on.

I have a friend who has a beautifully forested area on her property. You walk down the path and are quickly surrounded by canopies of tall pine trees. This miniature forest welcomes solitude. Going deeper you hear Japanese elms humming as breezes blow through their leaves. She goes to this special place each day to be embraced by soothing beauty. Her breathing slows, her heart quiets, her thoughts move into the background. She travels from the duress of the daily world to a healing peace. This is what we seek in meditation.

Meditation touches the mystical in man, the part of us that brims with metaphor and awe. Just as a yoga pose performed with clear focus on the breath brings steadiness and calmness, each meditation opens in us what has been clenched too long, held in pain and numbed to feeling. Meditation unties the ropes of sorrow, anxiety, depression and confusion that have bound us for so long. It is instrumental in exposing what we have hidden from ourselves. As we continue to practice, insights arise. The psychological and emotional pain that we have carried throughout our lives becomes lighter and fades. Life histories of suffering and want are released into calming seas. Here we are held like beloved babies.

Through meditation, we can develop a psychological and emotional immunity from those who project negative and aggressive unconscious feelings on us. A consistent meditator recognizes these individuals quickly and is able to deflect their toxic effects.

There is something both childlike and profound about doing a brief mediation in your bed at night. It is very still; there are no distractions. The darkness calls us to close our eyes and look inward. We hear and feel the breath gently moving in and out of our nostrils. We are receptive in this quiet darkness.

Some individuals prefer to meditate outdoors. The Buddha often meditated under a tree. He spent much of his long life walking and living in nature. He gave up the role of prince and the opulence of an easy surface existence to solve the issue of what causes human suffering. After much inner searching and experimenting, he discovered what he called the Middle Way. This is neither the extreme austerity of inflicted pain and severe self-denial nor the life patterns of self-indulgence and pleasure seeking.

One way of knowing that you are making headway with meditation practice is what happens when you skip several days or a week. You feel different. Your mind is not as steady; you are not as capable of pulling back your projections; you are more caught up in the persistent voice of the ego. You become irascible, angry, confused, perplexed, annoyed and psychologically off-center. These messages are telling you to return to your meditation practice.

How to Meditate

Before you start meditating, make sure you are physically comfortable. I find that putting a shawl around my shoulders creates a feeling of privacy that helps me to concentrate. Close your eyes and focus your inner gaze slightly above the point between your eyebrows, the spiritual eye. Let your eyes rest there. This position holds your concentration and keeps you from falling asleep. Take three deep, slow breaths (diaphragm, belly, chest) through the nose. Hold your breath at the top. As you exhale through the mouth, notice the release of tensions throughout your body. Then begin observing your breath moving in and out at the tip of your nostrils. The "in" breath is cool; the "out" breath has been warmed by your body. Focusing on the breath in this way helps you to keep your attention on the present moment.

CONSISTENCY IS THE KEY

Consistency, not the length of the mediation, is what matters most in making your practice an integral part of your daily life. Choose a time of day that works for you. The practice of meditation is a process and is individual to each person. Be patient with yourself and nonjudgmental. Developing the habit of mediation forms slowly, in your own time.

One monk I know gave a talk about wading gently into the practice of meditation. He suggested starting with mini meditations of thirty seconds, one minute, two minutes, followed by a quiet resting period. These short meditations strengthen the capacity for learning to practice stillness. His focus is on the devotional quality of meditation, not on the time involved. This monk has spent many years in ashrams in India undergoing strict training. He was alone in silence for long periods of time. Yet this human being of high consciousness tells his audience to take small steps with patience toward oneself.

The power of the practice accumulates over time. When you become more consistent with your meditation, it is ever-present somewhere in your mind. Consistent practice builds psychological and spiritual stability and stamina.

Getting Back on Your Horse

When you miss a day, weeks, months or years of meditation, it can be discouraging. We become critical of ourselves, believe that we have failed and are inclined to stop meditating. However, it is never too late to resume your meditation practice. The old advice to "get back on your horse" after you have been thrown applies to your return. There are no judgments to be made, no regrets, no guilt. Each time you resume your meditation practice the accumulated grace of your devoted and skillful actions returns to you a thousand fold.

Meditation Deepens Intuition

Meditation sharpens and enlarges our perceptions of reality while it dilutes and minimizes the forces of delusion. We are all susceptible to delusion. Delusion is an ego-based belief about the nature of reality.

Intuition does not require study or research. The more consistently we respond to the voice of intuition, the stronger our capacity to receive messages of truth becomes. The intuitive communicates in endless ways. It comes through as a clear voice that we don't recognize as our own, takes the form of a visceral feeling in the body or a clear inner knowing.

Not everyone recognizes the validity of intuition, so it is not always wise to share this knowledge. Most people will think you are jumping to conclusions or believe you are eccentric or strange. They do not understand the nature and truth of intuition.

Intuition protects us from human predators and is an endless creative tool. When we face a new project and are unsure of the first steps, intuition speaks. It can reveal itself in a complete product, like a book that takes shape quickly by itself or a piece of melody that insists on being written.

Working with intuition, be ready for surprises. We hear a message that comes into our minds, not in our words or style. This is a unique voice, not a hallucination or a delusion. It is direct truth.

On one occasion, I was driving my old car along a two-lane road. The car had a lot of mileage on it and I knew the time was coming soon when I would have to give it up. I needed to slow down to turn into a driveway. I stepped on the brake; nothing happened. I tried to change gears—nothing! My adrenaline rose. I felt trapped and helpless, bracing myself in a runaway car about to have an accident. Suddenly a voice said insistently: "Over the curb, over the curb, over the curb." That doesn't make any sense, I thought to myself. I argued with the voice. Then, in desperation, I went over the curb several times. The car slowed down. I felt my hand automatically reaching for the emergency brake and pulling it up. The car stopped in a spot perfectly aligned with the curb.

I am not mechanically inclined. I would never have thought to go over the curb. It was as if a hand took over mine and stopped the car for me. In this case, responding to my voice of intuition kept me from getting into an accident and hurting myself and others. I listened and acted upon the intuitive voice that told me exactly what to do. This resource is always with us. As you pay more attention to these communications, your capacity to tune into intuition expands and deepens.

Meditation isn't easy, but the benefits of opening yourself up and strengthening your intuition are worth it. The great spiritual teacher Paramahansa Yogananda speaks eloquently of the eternal power and resonant force of meditation:

> You may control a mad elephant;
> You may shut the mouth of the bear and the tiger;
> Ride the lion and play with the cobra;
> By alchemy you may learn your livelihood;
> You may wander through the universe incognito;
> Make vassals of the gods; be ever youthful
> You may walk in water and live in fire;
> But control of the mind is better and more difficult.

CHECKING YOUR PROGRESS:

- Briefly describe how your meditation practice is progressing.
- When you miss a day, week or month, how do you "get back on your horse?"
- What benefits have you noticed as a result of your meditation practice?
- Has your practice of meditation awakened your creative process? What have you noticed?
- How has your intuition become sharper and deeper since you have started meditating? Give a couple of examples.

CHAPTER 8

Evolution of the True Self: Becoming Whole

The spontaneous gesture is the True Self in
action. Only the True Self can be creative
and only the True Self can feel real.

—D.W. WINNICOTT

What can we gain by sailing to the moon
if we are not able to cross the abyss that
separates us from ourselves? This is the most
important of all voyages of discovery...

—THOMAS MERTON

THE TRUE SELF IS THE vital part of us we have inhabited since birth. It is the spontaneous core within that is free to express feelings and thoughts, to experience and create beauty as unique individuals. We inherited the gift of the original self. We are entitled to reclaim our natural selves and must do this to become whole. Our goal throughout life is to recognize, develop, nurture, express and manifest the fullness and richness of our inheritance.

Working through the process of separation and individuation from parental conditioning strengthens the original true self. As the true self expands and deepens, destructive psychological repetitions from the past lose their influence and power. Creative energies are set free. The rivers of the imagination bubble and surge with renewed life, the reticent heart opens, the restless mind quiets.

THE BABY SELF

It is difficult to remember that we were all babies and small children. We have lost touch with our baby selves— the belly breathing, expressive, marvelous beings we were designed to be. One of my favorite experiences is communicating with babies. I am fascinated by their individuality; awareness levels; openness; pure vitality; penetrating, unblinking gaze and the emotional connection they make with you. Happy babies express themselves with their whole bodies. They kick, squeal, gurgle, arch their tiny backs, coo, wiggle and giggle. Young babies have a sense of humor. When you smile and speak to them, they sense that you are making special contact. They reciprocate with a special smile. When we communicate with babies, we feel the full force of the pulse of life. We share the baby's ecstatic state that ignites in us the primordial joy of being alive.

One of the best ways is to practice being in the moment is to get in touch with the baby inside of you that is waiting to be set free. In this state, you are neither thinking about the past nor anticipating the future. Tune into your body; feel and enjoy its aliveness.

Like the baby, we need to learn how to play with our toes again. There is a yoga pose called Happy Baby, *Ananda Balasana* in Sanskrit, that you do lying on the mat on your back with your feet skyward. You reach for the sides of your feet and open your hips. This is a great move that brings soothing and contentment.

We were created to live fully in our bodies, feeling pleasure and strength. The healthy person experiences a flow of energy throughout the body. The happy child radiates unrestrained energy. He is uninhibited, spontaneous and unselfconscious. The baby's sounds, movements and gestures ebb and flow. He gets excited and kicks. His eyes light up and we see ourselves within them. Once a baby has locked on to you, his gaze stays with you. You have made a connection. He rewards you with a thousand-watt grin.

USING BREATH AND BODY TO HEAL
In the beginning, there was the breath. In Eastern traditions, for thousands of years, the uses of the breath in all

of its forms have been studied to understand and change consciousness and enhance deep contemplation.

The breath moves through every body system: circulatory, respiratory, endocrine, digestive, and excretory. The breath bathes every organ with its healing balm. It gently stretches the voluntary and involuntary muscles of the body, cleanses the blood and quiets the nervous system. Breathing brings fresh oxygen into the blood that nourishes and revitalizes the entire body and mind.

One summer night in northern Colorado near the continental divide, I watched the star-filled skies of the Milky Way with great wonderment. I was astonished and awed by the brilliance and enormity of their presence. I had never seen this light show. Yet each night the star- and planet-filled skies shine whether we are there to view them or not. This reminds me that the force and reality of the healing process through the breath is always occurring. Minute changes are taking place in the body and mind that are creating the conditions for wellness. Like the stars that are ever-present, steady healing is taking place through the sacred breath.

EXERCISE YOUR WAY

An essential part of healing is the reshaping of habits, attitudes and daily routines that add balance and structure to your renewed life. In the past, much of your time, energy and creativity were co-opted by the narcissist's demands, criticisms and cruelties. Whether we are the child, spouse or sibling of a narcissist, they have dictated our daily routines and schedules. This is especially true if we grew up under the control of a narcissistic parent.

Begin where you feel comfortable. Be realistic. What kind of exercise did you enjoy in the past? What appeals to you now? What gives you a feeling of well-being and strength? Many of us don't say to ourselves, "I can't wait to exercise." Rather we know we are at a starting point and have made a decision to exercise consistently to become healthier and build strength and physical confidence.

Walking is an excellent all-around exercise. As you walk you observe everything at close range—trees, grasses, wildflowers, sprouting seeds, thick hedges, tangled weeds, mud, flowing water, abandoned spider webs, tiny nets of insects and birdsong. With each step you become more grounded to the earth and gain a sense of stability.

Cardiovascular exercise in the form that works for you—stationary cycling, elliptical machines, rowing, climbing, walking, running—releases endorphins, powerful brain chemicals that boost the immune system, help us sleep better naturally, give us more energy and have a profound effect on stabilizing our moods. Cardiovascular exercise oxygenates the entire body, relaxes frayed nerves, and slows down obsessive thoughts. After cardiovascular exercise the calming part of the nervous system, the parasympathetic, takes over. It communicates to the body, mind and psyche that feelings of deep relaxation are now active throughout every neuron and cell.

CALMING THE BODY AND MIND

Learning to breathe diaphragmatically and practicing it regularly maintains a consistent feeling of security and steadiness throughout the body, mind and psyche. Most people breathe high in their chest, which does not engage the parasympathetic nervous system. Trained opera singers breathe correctly, through the diaphragm. Without straining their voices they reach the back row of any concert hall without a microphone or sound system.

Gently press your diaphragm with the flat of two or three fingers. Inhale and feel a resistance between your fingers and your diaphragm. Exhale and release the air from your lungs. You determine the counts as you inhale and exhale. Practicing diaphragmatic breathing with consistency activates the parasympathetic nervous system, putting your body and mind in a state of calmness and restoration.

The body is not separate from the mind and psyche. We are part of a seamless, interdependent package. The body naturally moves toward health and wholeness when we provide the necessary conditions. These nutrients are whole fresh food, healing sleep, a form of meditation that works for you, cardiovascular exercise and a regular practice like gentle yoga that strengthens all of the body's systems.

HEALING BODY AND MIND WITH GENTLE HATHA YOGA

Hatha yoga is a 5,000-year-old ancient healing practice created and developed in India. It uses a series of specific body postures, called *asanas* in Sanskrit, that the student approximates through concentration on the breath and mental focus.

Regular practice of hatha yoga fortifies the immune system, improves digestion and is helpful for getting quality sleep. The *asanas* create a more flexible spine, increase blood circulation, cleanse toxins from the body, strengthen nerves and tone the endocrine glands including the adrenals, thyroid, parathyroid, pineal, pituitary and thymus. Hatha yoga reinvigorates the body systems: the internal organs, the heart, the vascular system, the digestive system, the intestinal tract and the skeletal muscular branch including bones, joints, muscles and tendons.

When practicing yoga, remember there is no perfect pose. What you are able to do one day will be different the next. It is making the effort and doing your best, without judgment, that matters.

Performance is not the purpose of yoga. Yoga takes place deep inside you. Some people prefer to do their practice alone and find comfort in solitude. Others attend classes with well-trained teachers who are knowledgeable about the postures and their purposes, who have dropped their egos and are devoted to helping their students as a group and individually. If you are planning to take classes, appraise the teacher carefully and make sure he or she is devoted to the practice of yoga. Yoga has become very popular these days and there are teachers who aspire to be instant gurus with devotees and have a power and money motive. Listen to your intuition when choosing a yoga teacher.

Practicing yoga consistently increases your powers of concentration. When you are working with a pose, your mind focuses intently on each breath and movement. The capacity to use the mind to concentrate in this way accumulates and becomes stronger and more natural to your inner being. We bring our yoga practice into our daily lives and with it, increase one-point focus and deepen a capacity for inner peace.

FREEING BLOCKED EMOTIONS

Emotions flow naturally when we are consciously aware that we are living in our bodies. Many individuals have "forgotten" how to express their feelings. They learned early to freeze or deny their emotions as a result of parents' negative and punitive reactions to their spontaneity. Crying, laughing and expressing anger, regret and deep sadness were never allowed in these households. As a result, many individuals are emotionally frozen and numb.

Tight muscles in the neck, head and shoulders are a response to stress in the body and limit natural, full breathing. Many children learn to control their feelings by becoming accustomed to shallow breathing. This is the result of constant fear and apprehension due to parents who are cruel, demanding, cold and dismissive. Children who are subject to chronic psychological trauma learn very early to conceal their feelings from their parents and themselves. They tighten their bodies, and as a result they breathe in a shallow manner. This is survival breathing. They say to themselves: "Don't make a sound or say a word. You are in danger. Hold your breath, don't move." These messages are internalized in the body and mind and become part of an automatic reaction to perceived danger.

The first step in unblocking emotions is to recognize that they are being denied, numbed down or tightly controlled. The next move is to give yourself permission to let your human side be expressed, whether this means crying, laughing. Allowing yourself to do this without shame or self-recrimination is the beginning of wholeness.

Those who have lived under the tyranny of a narcissistic parent or spouse have conditioned themselves not to cry. They were taught that crying is degrading and an indulgence of the weak. I have seen clients make the greatest efforts to avoid crying. The eyes become liquid and start to fill. Just before the spilling of tears, there is a tightening in the body and face, a chronic habit learned from childhood to stop them. Crying is not shameful; it is human and essential to your healing. When we cry, it activates the parasympathetic nervous system, the part of us that is designed for open expression and healing release.

RHYTHM AND DANCE

Our bodies express emotion through spontaneous movement and sound. The more often you let go and move, dance, sing or chant, the more quickly and deeply these essential elements of your natural self become a part of your renewed identity and add joy to your life.

Dancing to music is an activity that many of us have ignored since childhood or never done. Some families don't have an environment of music or dance in their homes. If you missed those years, do it now. Find music that speaks to you in the language of the heart and celebrates imagination and beauty. Dancing in this way is not cerebral; it is joyous abandonment. Let the beat and melody carry you. Feel your body loosen. Enjoy your sensuality. Throw in some steps that you know, or improvise. Dancing breaks down the barriers of the obsessive thinking mind. When we move to music, we respond to a deep inner longing to put gesture to our feelings, to express ourselves freely through our bodies, to be taken both away and within: away from the constriction of our daily lives and within the joy and freedom of the melody and beat that calls us.

We are born to rhythm. In the womb the baby hears the beat of the mother's heart long before birth. We are destined from the beginning to recognize and respond to music. We are born to move, dance and flow with music.

Music carries us to psychophysiological states: joy, sadness, awe and calm. We respond to the music without thinking of our next moves. We are urged on by the rhythms that speak to us in their own language. Prehistoric cave paintings like those found in the Magura Cave in Bulgaria show men and women dancing. Our response to the beat and capacity to move rhythmically have been a part of man's evolution, going back 1.5 million years.

HUMOR: THE GIFT THAT SAVES US

Vital to the expression of the real self is rediscovering your sense of humor. Humor is spontaneous and makes life tolerable and triumphant. Humor shifts our chronic moods and smoothes the sharp corners of our pain. When we laugh and are carried away by whimsy and silliness, we lighten our emotional burdens. In this state, life is dynamic, rich and unbounded. An expression used about someone who is reeling with laughter is that they cannot contain themselves. We are spilling over, ecstatic, out of our narrow minds.

Humor is a precious gift. Its source is the unconscious mind. Openness to the unconscious stokes the richness of our humor. The more we activate humor, the deeper and more expansive it becomes. When we share laughter with others we create a bond. Humor is a life companion. The more you engage your humor, the easier it is expressed. We are born with a great potential for humor—use it to the fullest.

When you are freed from the narcissist, the world of humor opens. There are no limitations or boundaries. In darkest times, human beings call upon humor to breathe life back into them.

Humor and laughing have beneficial effects on the body and mind. They lower blood pressure, have a cleansing effect on the lungs, relax all the systems of the body, boost the immune system, protect the functions of the heart and lessen depression and anxiety. When we are laughing, our nervous system is in the parasympathetic mode—the relaxation switch is turned on.

Humor enlivens the entire body and mind. It lifts us up out of our personal life histories. We ascend to a delightful reality where we are fully ourselves, completely alive. The term "losing it" is perfect when we talk about the laughter contagion that takes place, especially between friends. The two of you look at one another and something starts to roll and gain momentum. You feed off of one another's quips and observations. Laughter builds into a spontaneous flow, a series of inevitable waves. The effects of laughter linger and heal us. When we laugh with abandon, we forget who we thought we were and become who we are.

DOWN TIME

Everyone is entitled to rest, solitude, reverie and repose, but most people today don't allow themselves any down time. They are rushing, driven and multitasking. Being heavily scheduled is prized in a society in constant movement. There are no moments to spare, even to talk with a friend. When you meet with one of these whirling dervish types, you are keenly aware that the person across from you is counting every minute, thinking only of the next event in his crowded schedule. He is not present and engaged. His engine is running. Uncommunicative and psychologically unavailable, he cuts you off to make a quick exit.

Whatever happened to down time? Some of the most creative and productive human beings spend segments of their days and evenings in a quiet, calm, unstructured environment.

One of the best venues for down time is being with nature. Immersing ourselves in its beauty and mysteries saturates our senses and offers boundless access to creativity

In the Western world, rest and sleep are undervalued. Overachievers who sleep less are praised for their drive and accomplishments. We ask ourselves: "Why can't we be like them?" "They perform at the highest levels." "What's the matter with me that I need so much sleep?" Don't get caught up in this fallacious thinking. Sleep is blessed. It keeps us physically, mentally, psychologically and emotionally healthy. When we sleep, all the organs of the body are restored, cleansed and fortified.

We dream every night. Most of us don't remember our dreams. Whatever is on our minds, in our emotions and psyche, bubbles up from the unconscious as we dream. Dreams are superb messengers. They tell us exactly where we are psychologically and emotionally. Each person has his own dream language that is filtered through his unconscious. Learning to decipher your dreams is invaluable. Dreams are symbolic, offering powerful images that cannot be imagined in our waking state, a collage of life events, experiences long forgotten beyond the locked door of repression. These night dramas are conjured up by the writer of the script, the dreamer himself.

THE HEALING POWER OF THE PARASYMPATHETIC NERVOUS SYSTEM

The autonomic or visceral nervous system is involuntary and not under conscious control. The functions of the autonomic nervous system include respiration, diges-tion, salivation and perspiration. Within the autonomic nervous system are the parasympathetic, sympathetic and enteric nervous system, which controls the gastroin-testinal system. The sympathetic nervous system mobi-lizes the body quickly into the fight-or-flight survival mode essential to maintain life. The parasympathetic has the role of dampening down the body and mind and oscillating into a state of calmness, security and peacefulness.

When the sympathetic system is in operation, the body prepares for the battle to survive, to live or die. This is built into the design of the nervous system so that when we are threatened we have the internal resources to either defend ourselves or flee to safety. Many people are in some stage of fight-or-flight. They are apprehensive, hypervigilant and suspicious. If the sympathetic pattern predominates, the individual is at the mercy of strong feelings of danger and immi-nent disaster. This is manifested as intestinal distress, muscle tension, rapid and shallow breathing, racing thoughts and adrenaline rushes. When these survival symptoms become chronic, they enervate and exhaust the body and mind. Those who have spent too much time on the raw edge of the sympathetic nervous system with narcissists—spouses, parents, siblings— need help dialing into the parasympathetic mode and finding a reservoir of relaxation and restoration.

All healing begins by consistently accessing the parasympathetic nervous system. This is a state of letting go as you bathe in physical and psychological security, peace and body and mind grounding. This calm waking state is natural and built into our being.

In the parasympathetic you float down a gentle river, letting the waters take you in a direction of their own. You feel receptive to the freedom and ease you're experiencing. As you consistently visit this state of calm, the healing of psyche, body and mind accumulates and moves forward at a steady pace.

One of the immediate ways of healing the body and mind is through the Chinese medical science of acupuncture. An ancient healing practice that goes back 4,000 years, acupuncture is based on balancing qi, a vital, universal energy in all living things. During acupuncture, fine needles are inserted into specific points called meridians, which are intricate pathways that move blood and qi. The skillful placement of needles balances all of the body systems: endocrine, nervous, cardiovascular, excretory, immune, digestive, respiratory, reproductive and skeletal muscular. When practiced expertly, acupuncture reawakens the parasympathetic nervous system, the great healer within us. Our true natures are reborn as we rest in quiet, calm, protective and restorative waters.

Acupuncture creates balance and harmonizes the body and mind in an elegant, subtle way. Over time, the positive effects of acupuncture profoundly affect all the body systems and create new pathways of healing. It strengthens weak organs and quiets those that are overworked and inflamed.

Acupuncture allows us to bathe in the parasympathetic, where there are no boundaries, no division of seas in the body and mind, only the deepest blue of calm and solace. Returning and staying in this "blue zone" creates neuronal pathways where hope arises and meets insight. You become the vessel through whom deep knowing and grace flows; the pain and burden of your personal history fades. When this first happens, it can be startling. You have been worried, frightened, on edge and hypervigilant since you were a small child. This has been part of your identity. As you go deeper with each healing experience, you begin to shed this painful burden. Unfettered and free, you are lifted by a gathering peace.

In the parasympathetic, some individuals hear words of healing insight. Others see an array of colors. The parasympathetic state is unique to each individual. As you build psychophysiological strength and stamina, you come into closer contact with your real self.

The work worth doing on Earth is acknowledging and dealing with our psychological and emotional survival patterns etched into the psyche. This conditioning of trauma and deprivation does not repair itself. We deal with it through a process of revelations and intuitions, by cracking the survival messages and releasing long-held, blocked emotions and by accessing the parasympathetic nervous system. Doing this work, we let go of what we had to believe about ourselves in order to survive, release it and begin a new cycle of evolution, a return to our true, original selves.

CREATING BLUE ZONE ISLANDS

An innovative way to immerse yourself in the parasympathetic nervous system is to create "blue zone islands" within your living space. Surrounding yourself with variations of the color blue activates a soothing response inside of us. Blue, in its limitless varieties, embraces us with exquisite healing beauty.

When we lie down and look up at the sky, we feel ourselves drifting to a quieter place. We marvel at the subtle changes in shades of blue as the moments roll by. From the beginning of the day to the darkest night, blue is there above us. Ocean blues, in the shallows and depths, are infinite.

Let yourself flow with the colors of blue that touch you deeply and evoke feeling and sensations of peace and wonder—robin's egg, periwinkle, turquoise, lapis lazuli, denim, sapphire, Prussian blue, azure, cerulean, cobalt, hydrangea, moonstone, cornflower, teal. Bring blue zone objects into your daily experience. Surround yourself with collections of colored stones, shells, glass beads, woven fabrics and tapestries, objects that have meaning to you alone. Put them in special places in your living space—on tables, in the kitchen, in the bathroom, on window sills, by your bedside—anywhere you can pause for beauty.

Another blue island zone activity is designing a wall that is devoted to prints, paintings, tapestries, collages, scarves and shawls, objects that you find calming, inspiring and beautiful.

YOUR UNCONSCIOUS LEADS THE WAY

The unconscious is mystical, innovative, creative and mysterious. Most people spend their lives reacting to their unconscious motivations, memories, impulses and passions rather than becoming consciously familiar with this rich source.

Dreams gestate and are born in the unconscious while we sleep. Each dream is as unique as the dreamer. Dreams convey vital messages to us. They warn us to change our entrenched, negative thought and behavior patterns. Many of us have recurring dreams that are vitally important in telling us what we are unable to understand or confront in our waking lives. They make every effort to rouse us out of delusion while we are asleep. There are precognitive dreams that foretell the future. The unconscious is dynamic, mysterious and filled with creative abundance.

Recently I had a nightmare. When I awakened, it was very difficult for me to shake the powerful grip of its vivid bizarre characters, catastrophic events and feelings of helplessness. The dream images persisted in my mind, and despite knowing I was awake I believed the dream was real. As I worked with the aftermath of the dream, I finally "got" something I had never understood. I knew on a gut level what the great spiritual masters tell us about the power of delusion over the human mind. They have provided us with specific practices like meditation to help us wake up from the dream of life to the truth. As difficult as it was for me to separate from my nightmare images, it is so much harder for me to sever myself from the delusion of the world and to become fully "awake." Nightmares, although terrifying, provide us with essential messages from the unconscious that tell us the truth about our inner selves. Doing consistent spiritual practice keeps us from falling asleep beneath the veils of delusion.

HOLDING THE LOTUS FLOWER OF TRUTH

Buddha uses the metaphor of the lotus flower that has its beginnings in muddy waters to explain how we can overcome the delusions of the world. Born into a world of delsusion, we, like the lotus flower, through consistent spiritual practices like meditation, fulfill our ultimate purpose: to rise through the murky and treacherous waters of our personal life histories.

In Sanskrit, the word *padma* means lotus. The lotus is a magnificent flower of many colors: white, pink, red and blue. The flowering of the lotus begins in muddy roots and grows up through the water to rise with great beauty. In Buddhism, the lotus symbolizes the soul's journey toward enlightenment. Rising eight to twelve inches, the lotus is like the soul that has been purified.

Knowing and speaking the truth is a spiritual blessing and a worldly curse. If you are clear and truthful, you don't have a lot of friends. Knowing and speaking the truth about human nature is part of your destiny if you are to evolve as a human being. Do you want to be popular and adored, or do you choose to be someone who speaks the truth? Truth glides through the fingers of most men like the sea that washes rocks smooth over millions of years, but knowing, holding and telling the truth is the essence of your evolution as an individual. No one, not even the most powerful or so-called holy men and women on Earth, can deny or take away the immutable truth from you.

You will find certain individuals, jewels of uncommon brilliance, who are special people that come into your life. These are the keepers of your soul, the ones who abide with you and help you to continue to grow. You, in turn, are ever present for them. In a vast sea of spiritual murkiness, you dove deep enough and far enough to reach out, touch and place the luminous jewels of great souls into your hands and heart.

THE HEALING MOMENT

As spiritual practice becomes a regular part of your life, you view others through a clearer lens. You become acutely aware of their suffering, longings, impediments and obstacles, and how you can reach out to them. The healing moment occurs when the receptivity of the individual in need merges with the open heart and insight of the other. In this moment, the impediment, the heavy obstacle that obstructed the life of the individual in need, loosens. The individual is released from his painful psychological wounds and transcends to free himself, becoming more authentic and alive. There is a sharing of the deepest humanity and heart-centered energy by both spirits. We invest ourselves in lifting up those whom we hear calling our name. Freed now, they touch the ground of their being and experience a healing peace.

UNEXPECTED VISITATIONS

How often in your life have you been visited by family members and friends who have left the body? The incidents are as varied as the individual who is contacting us.

Sean, a clairvoyant friend of mine, has had several visits from the ghosts of those who are dear to him. Grieving the loss of a beloved older male friend, he tells this story. Sydney was a highly successful, generous fellow, full of joie de vivre. He lit up every event he attended with his lively sense of humor, his zest for life and his deep affection for his friends. Once a week Sydney attended a regular poker game. He was prompt—he arrived every Friday night at exactly 9pm. On a hot summer evening one week after his death, everyone gathered to play poker. At precisely 9pm, my friend Sean stood near the closed front door. It automatically opened, ushering in a sudden rush of frigid air. A presence lingered in the atmosphere and Sean immediately knew that Sydney was visiting those he cherished. A week later, the same phenomenon was repeated. At 9pm the closed front door opened automatically, followed by an updraft of ice-cold air. Sydney had returned once more to communicate his deep affection. Sydney's visitations have had a powerful healing impact on my friend, and he recalls them with gratefulness, amusement and the comfort that Sydney transcended this life and is at peace.

Sean had another visitation in the company of Dominick, a man who had recently been widowed. Sean had known Dominick for several years. They were friends and fellow chess players who met weekly at the park. In the last several months, Dominick's wife Sarah had become very ill. Because she could not afford medical care in the United States, she returned to her family in another country. Dominick, who loved Sarah deeply, was unable to accompany her home due to lack of money. When Sarah reached her destination, she was desperately ill and died soon after her arrival. A week after her death, Sean was visiting his grieving friend Dominick at his apartment. They were sitting on the sofa talking. Sean noticed that the inside door to the living room was opening. He motioned to Dominick. Immediately a blast of frigid air came through them.

Sarah had come to visit and reassure her husband and Sean that she had successfully made the transition from this life to the next. This was a validation to Sean and Dominick that Sarah had reached her new destiny.

Soul Meetings

Soul meetings take place when we don't expect them. The key to cultivating soul meetings is your familiarity and communication with the deepest parts of yourself and your openness to others. We meet souls all the time. To recognize the soul of another person, we move to the part of our inner self that is operating when we are meditating or in deep concentration. There is an opening to the inner core of the other person.

Meeting a soul, you attune yourself to that person on a spiritual and psychological level. They feel your empathy. In this interchange, the souls meet and healing takes place. Soul meetings ease chronic psychological pain and trauma and renew hope. When we experience a soul meeting, we both receive and leave a spiritual imprint on the souls with whom we communicate.

The Universe Within

The outward universe of billions of galaxies thrills us.

Familiar names are Andromeda, our closest neighbor that can been seen on moonless nights with the naked eye; Sombrero, a glorious sphere like billions of pave diamonds; and Pinwheel, a galaxy of rose, blue and lavender, hurtle through space. We have access to both the external and internal universe.

Within us is the vastness that inhabits our inner space. This is the dwelling of the true self and the soul. The inner self is boundless and ever evolving like our earthly home in the Milky Way.

We spend our lives expanding and deepening the true self. We learn to recognize the special gifts given to us at birth. This knowledge comes to us through learning how to quiet the mind and become more awake. These creative gifts are unique to each individual. As you practice calming the nervous system, you become more aware of your inborn creativity. As we loosen the psychological knots that have bound us, we are set free to fulfill our destinies and use all of our spiritual and creative energies. As we evolve, we grow and deepen in insight, wisdom and empathy. There is an endless flow of grace that moves effortlessly through us when we rest in the universe within our true selves.

CHECKING YOUR PROGRESS:

- How are you getting in touch with your delightful baby self?
- Give an example of how you are using your breath to relax your body and mind (meditation, diaphragmatic breathing, gentle hatha yoga).

- Describe a soul meeting you have had recently or in the past.
- How do you feel when you are experiencing the parasympathetic nervous system?
- Recall a dream that has special meaning to you.
- What role does listening to your favorite music have in your healing process?

THANK YOU FOR READING MY BOOK. I HOPE YOU ENJOYED THE BOOK AND FOUND IT HELPFUL. IT WOULD BE MUCH APPRECIATED IF YOU WOULD LEAVE A REVIEW ON THE SITE WHERE YOU PURCHASED THE BOOK.

CHAPTER 9

Recovery Journal: Observing Your Progress

THIS CHAPTER IS YOUR CREATION and companion as you recover and rediscover your true self. The process of healing is not a straight line. There are forward movements, plateaus and back steps. These are all part of the intricacies and mysteries of the healing process.

In the journal you dialogue with yourself and discover fresh creative patterns of thought and feeling that are essential to your psychological and spiritual rebirth. As your healing progresses, you tap into a deep flowing reservoir of creative and psychic energy. You are adding newly born chapters to your life as you pursue the path of healing, wholeness and transformation.

DAILY WRITING PRACTICE

Spontaneous writing is a creative, healing and spiritual experience that activates the riches of the unconscious and moves you toward psychological wholeness.

- Have you noticed specific themes, metaphors or changes in your style of writing as you have been practicing? Describe them.
- What have you learned about yourself from your writing practice?
- As you let go of your inhibitions and judgments, is it easier to sit down and face the blank page or screen? How has this process surprised you?
- What is it like to be in the rhythm of your writing flow?
- Have any new feelings emerged as a result of your writing practice? How are these feelings significant to you?

Remembering and writing about ourselves as children primes the creativity pump.

- When I was a little child, I loved to _____.
- When I was a kid, it scared me when _____.
- As a child, I loved to make up stories about _____.
- When I was a little kid, I liked to spend time _____

- Two of my favorite books from childhood are _____ and _____.
- As a child, I learned _____ from watching adults.
- When I felt sad or lonely, I would _____ to help myself feel better.
- I liked to pretend I was _____.
- I made up stories about _____.
- Two of my best memories are _____ and _____.
- My favorite outdoor activities and games were _____.
- When I got scared I would calm myself by _____.
- Did you have imaginary friends? If so, describe one of them.
- What was your relationship with the world of nature? What are your clearest memories of nature?
- Did friends share their secrets with you? What is it about you that they could trust?

QUIETING THE MIND

When we practice meditation consistently, our thoughts slow down and our bodies become relaxed and comfortable. When the mind is at peace, we feel calmly alert and steady. The power of consistent meditation accumulates in the body and mind and sheds the delusions of the ego.

- Describe one of your meditation experiences.
- When and where do you meditate, and how does this work for you?
- Explain how you are becoming less judgmental about your meditation practice.
- Are you noticing keener intuition as a result of meditating? Briefly explain.
- Has meditation improved your ability to focus and concentrate? Give an example.
- How has your practice had an effect on your creativity? Describe some of your experiences.

STRENGTHENING THE BODY

Cardiovascular exercise engages the entire body. It strengthens the immune system and produces endorphins in the brain, activating feelings of well-being and calm.

- What cardiovascular exercise(s) are you doing regularly?
- How do you feel after cardiovascular exercise? Calmer? Quieter inside? More alert?
- Do you have an increase in mental clarity? What are you noticing specifically?
- How do you feel physically stronger and steadier?
- Have you noticed any changes in your sleep patterns since you've been exercising? Give an example.

HEALING MOVEMENT: GENTLE HATHA YOGA

Gentle yoga strengthens the body and mind on every level: muscles, tendons, joints, organs and spine. Yoga relaxes the mind and the body through the use of the breath and postures called *asanas*. This ancient practice will help your concentration, focus and stamina as well as calming your nervous system.

- How does yoga affect how you feel physically, mentally, emotionally, psychologically and spiritually?
- How has breathing through the nose helped you to become calmer? Give some examples.
- Are you more flexible as a result of yoga practice? Where in your body do you notice these changes?
- Has your concentration and focus improved since you have been practicing yoga? What are your observations?
- Do you feel physically stronger since you have been practicing yoga? Give a few examples.
- How are you more mentally alert? How does yoga help you to stay in the moment?
- Is your balance steadier since you have been performing yoga poses? Describe your experience.
- How do you feel calmer inside as a result of your yoga practice? Describe briefly.
- Are you more in touch with your inner self since you have started your practice? Explain.

SOUL MEETINGS: HEALING COMMUNICATIONS

Soul meetings are a natural function of our humanity. A deep sharing takes place between individuals. You both understand and are understood on a profound level during these healing communications. Two souls that meet have an experience of mutual healing. They are joined in a psychological and spiritual embrace.

- How does your intuition help you to recognize a person who is open to speaking with you on a deep spiritual level?
- How do you define a soul meeting? Briefly describe one of your experiences and its meaning and significance to you.
- How does your practice of stilling the mind— meditation, gentle yoga, being with nature, etc.— help you to become more receptive to soul meetings?
- What surprises you about soul meetings?
- How do soul meetings bring you closer to experiencing your true self?
- What are the psychological and spiritual gifts you have received as a result of soul meetings?

ABOUT THE AUTHOR

LINDA MARTINEZ-LEWI, PH.D., IS A clinical expert on the narcissistic personality, a psychotherapist and author. She offers in-depth analysis of the individual and their family of origin, strategies and practices for those psychologically abused by toxic narcissistic personalities through her books::*Recovering and Healing After the Narcissist* and *Freeing Yourself From the Narcissist in Your Life*, international telephone consultations and global podcasts (The Narcissist in Your Life Podcast).

Her book *Recovering and Healing After the Narcissist* puts the emphasis on transforming destructive psychological patterns of behavior, thought and emotion, accessing the parasympathetic body/mind systems that are calming and restorative and lead to the evolution and rediscovery of the true self. Visit her website: www. thenarcissistinyourlife.com

NOTES

CHAPTER ONE

"Finding the center of strength..." May, Rollo. *Man's Search for Himself.* New York: W.W. Norton & Company, 2009. Print.

"Because the development of inner calm..." Salzberg, Sharon. *Real Happiness: The Power of Meditation.* New York: Workman Publishing Company, 2011. Print.

CHAPTER TWO

"Like a seed growing into a tree..." Jacobi, Jolande. *The Way of Individuation: The Indispensable Key to Understanding Jungian Psychology.* New York: New American Library, 1983. Print.

"Knowing your own darkness..." Jung, Carl Gustav. *The Collected Works of C.G. Jung, Volume 16: The Practice of Psychotherapy.* Princeton, NJ: Princeton University Press, 1966. Print.

"The Soul loves to meditate..." Yogananda, Paramahansa. *The Autobiography of a Yogi.* Los Angeles, CA: Self Realization Fellowship, 1998. Print.

CHAPTER THREE

"The Buddha gave conditioned existence a name..."
Das, Lama Surya. *Awakening the Buddha Within: Tibetan Wisdom for the Western World*. New York: Broadway Books, 1998. Print.

"A thing which has not been understood..." Freud, Sigmund. "Analysis of a phobia in a five-year-old boy." *The Standard Edition of the Complete Works of Sigmund Freud*. Vol. 10. Ed. James Strachey. London: Hogarth, 1953. 122. Print.

"To abuse or neglect a child..." Shengold, Leonard. *Soul Murder: The Effects of Childhood Abuse and Deprivation*. New Haven, CT: Yale University Press, 1989. Print.

"...An attempt at soul murder." Shengold, Leonard. Ibid.

"The Mother's Son." Rudyard Kipling. Poem from: Shengold, Leonard. Ibid.

CHAPTER FOUR

"You should write, first of all..." Lessing, Doris. *The Golden Notebook*. New York: Simon and Schuster,1962. Print.

"Actually, every time we begin..." Goldberg, Natalie. *Writing Down the Bones: Freeing the Writer Within.* Boston: Shambhala Publications, 1986. Print.

"I get melancholy if I don't [write]..." Trevor, William. "William Trevor Quotes." Goodreads. 5 April 2015. Web.

"...[a]n absolutely instinctive" writer. Allardice, Lisa. "William Trevor: A life in books." *The Guardian.* 4 September 2009. Web.

"As the surface of the seashore rocks..." Trevor, William. *The Story of Lucy Gault.* New York: Penguin, 2002. Print.

CHAPTER FIVE

"The creative artist and the poet..." May, Rollo. *The Courage to Create.* New York: W.W. Norton & Company, 1975. Print.

"I dream of painting..." Van Gogh, Vincent. *Dear Theo: The Autobiography of Vincent Van Gogh.* Ed. Jean Stone. New York: Plume, 1995. Print.

"The dream is a little hidden door..." Jung, Carl Gustav. "The Meaning of Psychology for Modern Man." *CW 10: Civilization in Transition.* 1933: 304. Print.

"The Shadow personifies everything..." Jung, Carl Gustav. *The Archetypes and the Collective Unconscious.* (London 1996).

"Human subtlety will never devise..." Da Vinci, Leonardo. *The Notebooks of Leonardo Da Vinci.* Vol 1. New York: Dover, 1970. Print.

"They have been here!" Eliette Brunel. Quote from: Thurman, Judith. "First Impressions: What does the world's oldest art say about us?" *The New Yorker.* 23 June 2005. Web.

"Gardening was something I learned..." Claude Monet. Quote from: Fell, Derek. *The Magic of Monet's Garden: His Planting Plans and Color Harmonies.* New York: Firefly Books, 2007. Print.

CHAPTER SIX

"The job of a friend..." Shain, Merle. *When Lovers Are Friends.* Toronto: Bantam Books, 1978. Print.

"...True friendship is a kind of singing." Merton, Thomas. *The Red Diary.* New York: Image Books, 1968. Print.

CHAPTER SEVEN

"Every time we become..." Goldstein, Joseph. *Insight Meditation: The Practice of Freedom*. Boston: Shambhala Publications, 1993. Print.

"While absorbed in meditation..." Ma, Sri Anandamayi. *The Essential Sri Anandamayi Ma: Life and Teachings of a 20th Century Indian Saint*. Delhi: Motlal Banarsi Dass, 2007.

The monks "had been chanting..." Alfred A. Tomatis. Quoted from: Wilson, Tim. "Chant: The Healing Power of Voice and Ear." *Music: Physician for Times to Come*. Ed. Don Campbell. Wheaton, IL: Quest Books, 1991. Print.

Om is a Sanskrit word that means *avati* or *rakuati*... Saraswati, Swami Dayananda. "The Meaning of Om." *Arsha Vidya Gurukulam Satsangs*. AVG Satsangs. 5 April 2015. Web.

"You may control a mad elephant..." Yogananda, Paramahansa. *The Autobiography of a Yogi*. Los Angeles, CA: Self Realization Fellowship, 1998. Print.

CHAPTER EIGHT

Winnicott, D.W. *The Maturational Processes and the Facilitating Environment: Studies in the Theory of Emotional Development.* New York: International Universities Press, 1985. Print.

"What can we gain..." Merton, Thomas. *The Wisdom of the Desert.* New York: New Directions, 1970. Print.

REFERENCES

Allardice, Lisa. "William Trevor: A life in books." *The Guardian*. 4 September 2009. Web.

Da Vinci, Leonardo. *The Notebooks of Leonardo Da Vinci*. Vol 1. New York: Dover, 1970. Print.

Das, Lama Surya. *Awakening the Buddha Within: Tibetan Wisdom for the Western World*. New York: Broadway Books, 1998. Print.

Fell, Derek. *The Magic of Monet's Garden: His Planting Plans and Color Harmonies*. New York: Firefly Books, 2007. Print.

Freud, Sigmund. "Analysis of a phobia in a five-year-old boy." *The Standard Edition of the Complete Works of Sigmund Freud*. Vol. 10. Ed. James Strachey. London: Hogarth, 1953. 122. Print.

Goldberg, Natalie. *Writing Down the Bones: Freeing the Writer Within*. Boston: Shambhala Publications, 1986. Print.

Goldstein, Joseph. *Insight Meditation: The Practice of Freedom*. Boston: Shambhala Publications, 1993. Print.

Jacobi, Jolande. *The Way of Individuation: The Indispensable Key to Understanding Jungian Psychology.* New York: New American Library, 1983. Print.

Jung, Carl Gustav. *The Collected Works of C.G. Jung, Volume 16: The Practice of Psychotherapy.* Princeton, NJ: Princeton University Press, 1966. Print.

Lessing, Doris. *The Golden Notebook.* New York: Simon and Schuster,1962. Print.

Ma, Sri Anandamayi. *The Essential Sri Anandamayi Ma: Life and Teachings of a 20ᵗʰ Century Indian Saint.* Delhi: Motlal Banarsi Dass, 2007.

May, Rollo. *The Courage to Create.* New York: W.W. Norton & Company, 1975. Print.

May, Rollo. *Man's Search for Himself.* New York: W.W. Norton & Company, 2009. Print.

Merton, Thomas. *The Red Diary.* New York: Image Books, 1968. Print.

Merton, Thomas. *The Wisdom of the Desert.* New York: New Directions, 1970. Print.

Phillips, Jan. *Marry Your Muse: Making a Lasting Commitment to Your Creativity.* Wheaton, IL: Quest Books, 1997. Print.

Salzberg, Sharon. *Real Happiness: The Power of Meditation.* New York: Workman Publishing Company, 2011. Print.

Saraswati, Swami Dayananda. "The Meaning of Om." *Arsha Vidya Gurukulam Satsangs.* AVG Satsangs. 5 April 2015. Web.

Shain, Merle. *When Lovers Are Friends.* Toronto: Bantam Books, 1978. Print.

Shengold, Leonard. *Soul Murder: The Effects of Childhood Abuse and Deprivation.* New Haven, CT: Yale University Press, 1989. Print.

Thurman, Judith. "First Impressions: What does the world's oldest art say about us?" *The New Yorker.* 23 June 2005. Web.

Trevor, William. *The Story of Lucy Gault.* New York: Penguin, 2002. Print.

Trevor, William. "William Trevor Quotes." Goodreads. 5 April 2015. Web.

Van Gogh, Vincent. *Dear Theo: The Autobiography of Vincent Van Gogh.* Ed. Jean Stone. New York: Plume, 1995. Print.

Wilson, Tim. "Chant: The Healing Power of Voice and Ear." *Music: Physician for Times to Come.* Ed. Don Campbell. Wheaton, IL: Quest Books, 1991. Print.

Winnicott, D.W. *The Maturational Processes and the Facilitating Environment: Studies in the Theory of Emotional Development.* New York: International Universities Press, 1985. Print.

Yogananda, Paramahansa. *The Autobiography of a Yogi.* Los Angeles, CA: Self Realization Fellowship, 1998. Print.

Made in the USA
Las Vegas, NV
17 January 2022

41651011R00089